The Cover Picture: Graduation Day RCSI-1961 - The graduates of the 1961 class, from left to right: Willie Hickey, Kelly McNeice, Brian Lane, Des McManus, Frank Cawley, Conor McLaughlin, Eugene McKee, Tom Lomas, and Neil O'Brien

DOC

Revelations of a Reluctant Yank
Studying Medicine Among the Irish

PUBLISHER'S INFORMATION

eBookBakery Books
Author contact: genem1@cox.net

Editing by Tracy Hart
www.editingwithhart.com
editingwithhart@gmail.com
Paperback and cover design by the eBook Bakery
www.ebookbakery.com
authorhelp@ebookbakery.com

ISBN 978-1-938517-16-7

ACKNOWLEDGMENTS

The author wishes to express his appreciation to Tracy Hart, whose editorial direction has been invaluable, and to Michael Grossman, who expertly shepherded passage of the manuscript through the publication process.

DEDICATION

To my Father, Mother, and Aunt Bertha

TABLE OF CONTENTS

Part II

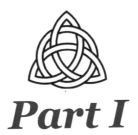

Part I

T he recollection of my days in Dublin and the medical school experience may be of little interest to anyone other than classmates and companions of the time. If others were to venture through these pages, however, I'd like to think they would gain some sense of the ambience that was Dublin and the College of Surgeons in the late 50s and early 60s.

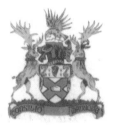

Crest of the Royal College of Surgeons

The impetus to commit pen to paper experienced a slow gestation. Many years ago, a classmate, Francis Ahearn, commented favorably on a short article I submitted to "Fleam," the College's alumni magazine. In her note, she suggested I expand the reminiscences touched on in the piece. For decades the thought kicked around in my head but various excuses kept it there. A diminished work schedule over the past two years freed up some time; I felt that if I was ever going to do it, now was the moment.

The capricious trip to Ireland in 1955, the start of the journey that eventually brought me to medical school, also initiated my flight from the cocoon of teen-age years to the precincts of adulthood. I hesitate to say that I reached maturity - as that continues to be a work in progress - but the first baby steps were taken, and significant strides have been made since.

I was exposed to a country whose existence, strangely enough, was only hinted at while growing up in my father's family, all of whom were Irish. St. Patrick's Day provided a reason for a corn beef and cabbage dinner and a green article of clothing, but the rest of the year passed without reference to our affiliation. When at various times I pressed for details of our family tree, the responses were vague. "Those people are gone; there's no need to bring them up," or "Grandma and Grandpa never talked much about them, so I really don't know." It seemed when the family arrived on America's shores a pledge was taken not to discuss the old country.

Also there was an inclination not to be associated with the negative notions some held of the Irish: a country of heavy drinkers with chickens in the kitchen and pigs in the parlor. My paternal grandmother, Ellen McCarthy, born in London of Irish parents, forever insisted she was English. Her daughter, my Aunt Bertha, red-haired with the map of Ireland etched on her face, when asked her ethnicity, till the day she died, replied: "English."

"Bertha," I would insist, "there's not a drop of English blood in you. How can you say you're English?"

"Because I am."

"I think you're a snob."

"Perhaps, but I'm an English snob."

I might add that on my mother's side of the family, also Irish, one encountered a different scenario. Any excuse was reason for a party – especially St. Patty's Day, the social equivalent of a Holy Day of Obligation. The celebration featured Irish stout or lager, shamrock badges, green-coned hats, and sentimental Irish songs, which as the evening wore on provoked teary-eyed nostalgia. And to remind all of the holiness of the day, the local parish priest was invited. The partiers would pause to follow the Father in a decade of the rosary. This invocation, usually accomplished later in the evening, evoked images of the wedding scene at Cana, about an hour or so after the arrival of the "good wine."

But in Ireland, I found a place and a people who, at that time in my life, suited me to the ground. A country whose topography - the moonscape of Connemara, the tropical oases that dot the south, the green-ruffled blanket of the Midlands, and the rock fortresses that guard the western shore - was as diverse as its populace.

I saw, firsthand, families who lived in crushing poverty, listened to conversations that bordered on the lyrical, shared their God-given sense of humor and irony, met women as beautiful as I've ever seen (but seldom knew), and worked with physicians whose skill I could only dream about. I knelt in pews with a community committed to their faith - who followed without question the dictates of an all-powerful, repressive Church. Consistently I was dazzled by the theater and the talent of its players, participated in their prodigal use of alcohol, sang their songs and danced their dance - and in some ways became as Irish as the Irish themselves.

I found that sometimes the sense of a people can best be illustrated by offering an example. One night, a year or so after entering the country, I happened to be enjoying a glass of stout at a public house in Ringsend, a hardscrabble collection of worn-out residences and tenements at the mouth of Dublin's Liffey River. Visible through the only window of the premises were a series of white lights, stretched like a necklace, along a curved pier at the end of which was a small lighthouse. The only other person in the place, besides the barman, was a man seated three stools away. His clothes were those of a worker: jacket and grease-stained trousers; a cap, its visor blackened, pushed back from a face sporting an irregular nose and a good four-to-five-day stubble of beard. Since most in that area worked the docks I assumed he did, and when we began our conversation he affirmed that was the case. As initial chats do, it traversed a variety of non-related topics: where to find the best pint in Dublin, English soccer, an up-coming rugby international, and an article by Myles na gCopaleen in the Irish Times.

A genial, non-argumentative sort, we had a pleasant exchange. As I prepared to leave, he abruptly asked, "Do you like poetry?"

"Can't say I do, maybe a little," I replied. "I have some favorites."

"Well, it's my hobby." He smiled. "I keep it quiet. My favorite is Percy French. Ever hear of him?"

"As a matter of fact," I answered, "I have a friend who recites a poem of his – "The Four Farrellys" - as something of a party piece."

Without hesitation, the man, with eyes closed, recited some of the verses.

When he finished, I added, "If you like that kind of thing, you should look up Robert Service, an Englishman who ended up in Canada. He wrote a lot of stuff like that, about the Yukon and the Arctic." I remembered enough of "Dangerous Dan McGrew" to give the man a feeling for Service's style.

The next thing I know, the barman was in front of us. "I've been listening to you two," he said. "I don't know any poetry but I remember in school reading a story I really liked." Then he started talking about the plot and it turned out to be *Treasure Island*. Soon he and my bar mate were going back and forth over the tale, each filling in the places the other had forgotten; the bar-keep was into it, as though he'd found a long lost toy.

I listened to them, in this little pub at the back end of beyond, talking about Long John Silver and seamen with parrots on their shoulders, and thought, *What the hell's going on here? It's like a meeting of the Ringsend Prose and Poetry Society.* But behind the flip remark was my increasing realization of the appreciation the Irish have for language. Though only the gifted can arrange syllables to create an "Isles of Innisfree," I'd never before seen (although my experience was limited), a general population so attuned to and facile with the spoken and written word - including the pedestrian crew in the pub that night.

16

For the remainder of the evening we sipped stout and talked "of many things, of shoes and ships and sealing wax, of cabbages and kings," and sampled from the repertoire of our poetic friend - who was beside himself in enjoyment.

When I remember Ireland, it's nights like that I remember most.

As this memoir unfolds, what will become increasingly apparent is the dominant role my aunt played in my life, certainly the main driver of things educational. Bertha never married (though she emphasized over the years that opportunities had been presented). No doubt she would have been a hand-full for any man. Intelligent (Masters Degree from Harvard) and with a haughty self- assurance, I couldn't imagine her being submissive to a husband (as scripture admonishes wives to be), or even to accept a marital status of parity - no matter how enamored she was of the gentleman. By the same token, few men would have tolerated the back seat they'd have been assigned in that marriage chariot. My arrival in her life gave her the opportunity to raise, mold, and influence the child she never had.

My aunt drew from a broad palette of interests. Musically inclined, she played fine piano. As a young kid I remember sitting beside her, turning the pages of the song sheet as we sang along together. "We Three, We're All Alone," was a particular favorite.

> "I walk with my shadow;
> I talk with my echo;
> But where is the one I love?"

Her love of big bands and dancing was passed on to me. The box step she showed me in the living room, I've taught my kids in the kitchen. Very athletic - skier, skater, swimmer, horseback rider - whatever the activity, she brought me along. Though, perhaps, not the most important person in her life, I certainly garnered a considerable portion of her attention.

I learned at an early age that to gain my aunt's acceptance

and favor, you needed to achieve some measure of excellence or be involved in something constructive. Opportunities arose in various guises: assisting the priest at Mass, shoveling out neighbors after snowstorms (for a fee), taking on a paper route, caddying (and creating a savings account to deposit all earnings). And most important of all: doing well in school. An exceptional report card or Honor Roll status brought the greatest accolades - golden boy status conferred until the next set of marks came out. Completing the fifth grade, Miss Houston designated me the smartest boy in the class for that year - the highlight of my academic career - and I was presented with a suitably inscribed book. That made for a wonderful summer, unfortunately not endless, as September and the challenges of sixth grade were soon on the horizon. (The story goes that Casanova was once asked how it felt to be known as one of the world's great lovers. In response he cited the disadvantage of his reputation - the constant pressure to perform well - and added, "In this business you're only as good as your last conquest." [The original Italian used a different word.] This aphorism would be apt regarding my situation with Bertha - but little else.)

A lifetime has elapsed since my student days in Ireland, and I was not optimistic that a coherent narrative could be fashioned. A journal, maintained through the summer of 1955, was discontinued when I returned to Ireland from France in September of that year. The events and conversations of the remaining years - with allowance for an occasional exaggeration - are as I remember them. Interestingly, while immersed in the process, the tide of recollection flowed easily; memories rekindled were leisurely savored the second time around. My hope is that this memoir will provide a similar experience for those who shared the day.

Neither the gray, brooding clouds nor the occasional splat of rain could dampen my excitement as I moved across the gust-ridden tarmac to board a Pan-Am Clipper. This trip, to gain acceptance to a European medical school, was my first out of the country. It was July 31, 1955, and I was catching an evening flight to Shannon, Ireland. The plane, four engines and propeller-driven, was being readied for the flight, its wing lights blinking a short distance away. An attractive stewardess led our small contingent across the runway. Nattily attired in a powder blue uniform and white blouse, her flight cap was secured by a thin scarf, also white, knotted beneath her chin. Forced on occasion to lean into the bursts of strong wind, she was a pleasant distraction as we made our trek.

A steel walkway was in place against the fuselage. After clanging our way up its slippery steps to the plane's entrance, we were greeted by another fine looking stewardess, her blue ensemble nicely complimented by blonde hair, gathered in a bun. After bestowing a welcoming smile and a Dixie-tinged "hello," she directed us to our seats.

I had a window seat and beside me, on the aisle, was an elderly priest. After introductions, he told me he was returning to his home in Ireland to retire, after serving for over thirty years as a parish priest at various churches in Massachusetts. His presence, I told him, provided a sense of security, and I hoped he'd be amenable to an emergency absolution, if it became necessary. The Father smiled, and without missing a beat, replied, "I'll absolve the whole plane if you could arrange to take up a collection beforehand."

The flight was smooth enough to allow for a few hours of fitful sleep. When nudged awake by a run of turbulence, I saw the sky had brightened. In the distance, a dark shape emerged which as I watched, lightened to purple and then a rose color as the sun broke over the horizon. Finally, there it was: the green of Ireland.

As we began our descent, the captain announced there was a problem with the landing gear, that touchdown might be a bit rough. The cabin became still as we made a series of passes over the airfield. The sun had swept clean the shadowed landscape, save for shrouds of mist which stubbornly clung to distant hills. A beautiful day was unfolding, much too lovely to be ruined by an awkward event.

My clerical seatmate seemed quite calm. "What do you think, Father," I asked, my voice having moved to a higher register. "Are we going to make it?"

He turned to me and smiled. "I can't believe the good Lord would cancel my retirement before it's even begun. I would be very upset with Him." He closed the breviary he was reading, put his glasses in a case and placed them both in a small brief-case beneath his seat. His only nod to possible nervousness: he removed his white collar, placed it on his lap and undid the top button of his black shirt.

The cockpit announced our final approach. As I watched, the widening green swath was replaced by the mudflats of a river. A jolt, less than expected, was followed by the sound of grinding steel on concrete. Grasping the armrest with sweaty hands and crouched forward as instructed, I watched chunks of rubber fly past the window as the plane shook violently. Abruptly, the screeching stopped and all was silent. Tension relieved and survival assured, applause erupted in the cabin. I shook Father's hand and told him how pleased I was that he had been on the flight.

A bus was driven out to take us to the terminal; on our way there it developed a flat tire. Many of us walked the remaining distance. Welcome to Ireland!! I hoped it wasn't an omen...

My undergraduate education had commenced in 1951 when I entered the College of the Holy Cross in Worcester, Massachusetts. My first choice was Providence College in Rhode Island, but my Aunt Bertha (with whom I lived along with my father), felt that Holy Cross would offer a better education, she being partial to the Jesuits ("the most intelligent order in the Church").

Shortly after my acceptance, Bertha and I sat down to finalize my courses for the upcoming year. My father left such matters to his sister, the "smart one," assuming her educated decisions would better serve my interests. My academic strengths never included the sciences, being much more comfortable with and interested in history, languages, and literature. I told Bertha I was looking forward to the B.A. English program which I thought had been agreed upon. Although appreciative of my preference, Bertha voiced her oft-repeated theme: even though the curriculum would be rewarding, it offered no meaningful (that is money-making), potential. Then the reason for the conversation became evident.

"I spoke with Dr. Sullivan last week," she began, (our family doctor and a graduate of Holy Cross), "and mentioned you'd be attending his alma mater. He was pleased for you, and when he asked what classes you'd be taking, I told him it was still being discussed."

"But," I interjected, "I thought we decided--"

"Let me finish, Gene. Naturally the doctor thought you should give pre-med a shot, and he went on extolling the program there. He also mentioned that you can do a B.A. along with the pre-med program – the best of both worlds...What do you think?" she asked.

Even at age 16 I knew where this was headed. "Bertha, I've

always been weak in the sciences. I have absolutely no interest in medicine."

"Look," she argued, "at least have a go at it. If it doesn't work, it doesn't work."

"I really don't want to, Bertha."

"I know you don't, but I think we'll give it a try."

I didn't respond. Once Bertha had made up her mind the decision was fixed - as in concrete - and my yelps of it being unfair would not affect her determination. Besides, she was footing most of the tuition bill; with her money on the table she controlled the dice.

"You do have one option," she added. "B.A. with Greek or Math."

I shrugged my shoulders. "Greek, I guess."

All of a sudden the allure that was college took a hit.

Throughout my years at Holy Cross I did well in subjects that captured my attention, but this never included science. Biology, physics, and various chemistry courses did not yield to my, arguably half-hearted, efforts. I regurgitated enough material to pass and continue in the program, but in my senior year it became evident that I would not receive the imprimatur of Father Busam, chairman of the premedical program, guaranteeing acceptance into medical school. He was quite candid in my exit interview. He said that while he would recommend me, it would not be with any degree of enthusiasm. Holy Cross had, as it does now, one of the best pre-med programs in the country, with 90 to 95% of its graduates continuing on to medical school. The good Father said he did not want to jeopardize the reputation of his program, and furthermore, thought that I should consider another field. I agreed completely.

At my graduation in June of 1955, I had in my possession a BA degree, a second lieutenant's commission in the United States Air Force, and I was wait-listed at two medical schools:

New York Medical College and Tufts University in Boston. I was scheduled to enter flight training in Texas, beginning in October, and was quite happy with my status. Although I enjoyed my days at the Cross (couldn't wait to return each fall), the pre-med experience had been painful, and I had no desire to continue the suffering in medical school.

An Unhappy Aunt

My parents, although separated for years, were similarly pleased that I had graduated from college: the first to do so in my mother's family. They both felt that the Air Force was an excellent opportunity, either as a career or for time to think about what to do with the rest of my life. The one person not pleased was my Aunt Bertha. She inferred, not too subtly, that I, at considerable expense, had wasted my years at Holy Cross. My aunt also felt, God bless her, that I could do better than fly around in an airplane, teach high school, or work for a local newspaper, the latter being what I really wanted to do.

Apart from everything else, however, medical school was a financial improbability: money was not available. My father was a maintenance man for a company in Providence, R.I., my mother worked as a live-in maid for a woman residing on the East Side of that city, and Aunt Bertha taught in the Providence school system. As for me, I only worked summers, and derived a good part of tuition for college as a fish cutter.

Resigned to my lot, I returned to Narragansett, R.I., a small coastal community at the southern end of the state. I reclaimed my job at the fishing co-operative and lived with my father and Aunt Bertha to wait the summer out.

At that point I felt the medical school expectation had been put to rest and was pleased with its resolution. As I should have known, this contentment didn't resonate with my doggedly focused, red-headed aunt. Out of the blue one evening, she announced her "Plan B."

"I've been asking around," she began, "and I'm surprised to find that some of the local doctors did their medical school work outside the country."

Here we go, I thought. *There's just no give-up in this woman.*

"I have a priest friend, Father Connelly," she continued, "who teaches at Boston College, but at one time taught in Dublin. I've contacted him and he will get in touch with a professor connected with University College Dublin...to inquire about admission possibilities and the acceptability of their medical degree in the U.S. It's worth a try, Gene."

The ensuing correspondence informed us that the medical class for 1955 had been filled, and furthermore, the professor felt quite certain that the UCD medical degree was *not* acceptable in the U.S. Aunt Bertha's ambition for me: thankfully thwarted.

A Fish Story

With that possibility eliminated, I returned to what was assumed to be an uninterrupted summer of cutting fish. The Co-Operative, located in Galilee, the local hub for commercial fishing, was a consortium of local fishermen. They banded together, acquired a central location for their catches, shared overhead, eliminated redundancies, and with the clout of the group, increased profit. Starting at age sixteen I had worked there summers, initially cleaning filets and preparing them for packing, then a step-up to skinner, and the final advancement to cutter. On any given day a cutter went through between two and three thousand pounds of fish, mostly flounder, earning a dollar for every hundred pounds of fish filleted. This translated to twenty-to-thirty dollars a day.

The trick in that business was the ability to maintain a sharp knife, a continual challenge. But apart from that, the boredom of standing from 8:00 a.m. until often 9:00 or 10:00 p.m. in the busy summer months, with just two half-hour breaks, was numbing. On the one day off, which in the fish business was Friday, I caddied. The checks I received from the Co-Op went directly into the bank, while I pocketed whatever I earned caddying at the Point Judith Country Club.

What social life I had was significantly restricted by the overpowering smell of fish I carried with me constantly, an odor totally resistant to soap, water or deodorant. The only people I felt comfortable going out with were other fish workers. Occasionally on a Saturday night a few of us went to a local dance venue, drank some beer, listened to Eddie Zack and his country ensemble, and tried to find a woman desperate to dance or with a really bad cold.

A Plan Is Hatched

It so happened that Aunt Bertha went on a European tour with a group of teachers that summer. Around mid-July I received a letter from her:

Dear Gene,

I've just finished a most interesting conversation with an American lady, attached to another touring group. During our chat I learned that her son was practicing medicine in New York, and like you, unsuccessful when he applied to American medical schools. But he contacted a British university, was accepted, graduated, and after passing an entrance exam, came back to the states. I think this is worth a try. Here's what I want you to do. . .

Her instructions were to take what money I had in the bank, approximately $800, book a flight to Ireland, and apply to schools there. Then, depending on how it went, continue on to Britain and perhaps even Europe. The only problem she foresaw was the possibility of having to learn another language.

At the time, it all sounded completely far-fetched. It was late July and fall classes were, in all probability, filled. In addition, I had no contacts abroad. I would be alone in a strange country with nothing to offer other than my diploma, a college transcript, and on occasion, a pleasant personality. However, standing at a bench eight to ten hours a day, with a dull knife and an endless stream of fish, made the thought of a summer tooling around the British Isles seem very attractive. I certainly wasn't driven by an overwhelming ambition to go to medical school.

Iquit my job at the Co-Op. The night before my departure, fellow workers threw a party for me at a local bar. I knew the singer there, Ginny Dailey, through her brother, another fish cutter. Later, when I drove her home, Fats Domino's "Ain't That a Shame" came on the radio. "It's a shame you're leaving," she said, and although I nodded in agreement, I was looking forward to the adventure. Leaving the country was a pretty exciting deal in my young life.

The following morning I took a bus to Providence. After checking my bag at the terminal, I walked up College Hill, past Brown University and the elegant Colonial mansions along Benefit Street, to 87 Williams St., to say goodbye to my mom. She worked there as housekeeper for Mrs. Metcalf, one of the landed doyennes of Providence society and also a very nice lady.

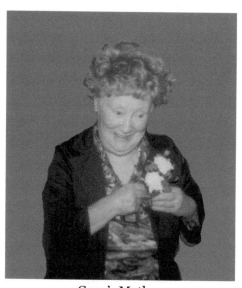

Gene's Mother

My mother was flabbergasted when I told her my plans. After the initial shock, came the torrent of questions: "How long will you be away?" "Where will you stay?" "How can I reach you?" None of which I could answer. My mother was a garrulous, out-spoken woman. Although she was not hesitant to express her feelings on whatever topic was under discussion, our relationship, sporadic and cordial, seldom if ever resulted in conflict. The occasional flares of irritation were short-lived and seldom directed at me. If we had interacted on a more consistent basis, or lived under the same roof, a more telling profile of our personalities would have certainly emerged. However, when upset, her voice rose, the tone more strident. And clearly, on that day, she was upset.

"Why didn't you let me know all this before now, Gene, the very day you're leaving?" She paused. "I'm still your mother. I should be involved in what you do. Was this Bertha's idea? I don't like being left out." Her clear, unlined face, assisted by a patina of unevenly applied make-up, had acquired a crimson hue.

I nodded. "It all came together quickly, Mom. And I didn't want to get you worried."

"And I will worry...in a foreign country by yourself."

"I'll probably be back in a few weeks. There's really no chance I'll get into a school at this late date. It's more of a summer vacation."

We chatted a while longer and she seemed more reconciled to the idea.

"You'll be careful, won't you?" She took my hand. "And you will write?"

"I will."

After a hug, she went into the adjoining room, returned with her handbag and gave me whatever cash she had.

Retracing my steps to Benefit Street, I left its affluent end and headed to Fox Point, located on the Providence River, comprised of working-class homes and light industry. India Point, the port, had been a major embarkation point for trade with India and China in the late 1700s and early 1800s. It was the American connection during the infamous triangle trade of slaves, sugar, and rum, between New England, the West Indies, and West Africa. Another neighborhood claim of distinction: it was the birthplace (on the "fourth of July") of singer/songwriter George M. Cohan, of "Yankee Doodle Dandy" fame, and where he launched his career.

My father worked in Fox Point for a medium-sized paper products company as a custodian. I found him in his "office" – a cluttered alcove in the basement of the building. Not expecting me, he was delighted we could say goodbye in person. He took me around and introduced me to all the "higher-ups" who looked at me somewhat askance when they learned I was off to Europe to find a medical school. However, they were enthusiastic for my success and wished me well. Little did they know that my motivation had nothing to do with medicine and everything to do with a desire to remove myself from the fish business.

We said our goodbyes on the sidewalk outside the building.

"I'm going to miss our swims, Gene," he said and smiled. "And I'll have no one to beat playing high, low, jack."

"I'll be gunning for you when I get back."

"You'll be in my prayers," he added quietly, shaking my hand.

"I know, Dad," I replied, as I knew I always was.

Walking back to the station I couldn't help but reflect on how different my parents were in personality, temperament, and style (and which of them I'd be most like). Curious how those differences had apparently been of little concern, at least for awhile, some seventeen years before. Despite my many attempts to learn the reason for the abrupt split (literally within weeks of my birth), it was never divulged. I would like to think that, if in a similar situation, I would have made more of an effort to hold the marriage together. But as the heart has its reasons, they had theirs. More unfortunate, sad really, was that neither one (at least to my knowledge), had ever enjoyed a romantic relationship since their separation.

At the terminal, I reclaimed my bag, boarded a bus and was off to Logan Airport in Boston.

Relieved and thankful to be on Erin's green sod, our group made its way across the tarmac to the terminal. The air was crisp, with winds sweeping in fresh from the Atlantic. Blue sky was marked with puffs of cloud forming over the coast; in the distance, I could see green fields dotted with cattle. Like postcards I had seen, Ireland was just as I imagined it would be.

The plan was to spend my first night in Cork city, a large seaport situated at the mouth of the river Lee, in the south-west corner of the country and where University College Cork was located. An airport bus brought me to the nearest city, Limerick, where train connections to Cork were available. Since it was Sunday I wanted to go to Mass; the train schedule obliged, offering an early afternoon departure.

I found a service being held in a large stone church in the center of town. As I checked out the congregation I made the rather astute observation that everyone looked the same--Irish. In a church, or any public place in the United States, you see a mixed bag of ethnicities. Here everyone had a basic similarity: big, broad men with white foreheads and ruddy, weather-beaten faces, most clad in a shirt and dark jacket with a loosened tie. The women wore long dresses, many with shawls, some whose complexions were pale and unlined, others looked as swarthy as the men's. Many of the older women were saying the rosary. On the altar stood two recently scrubbed altar boys and a bespectacled priest speaking in a language which I could only presume to be English. During the course of a barely comprehensible homily, thanks were given for the safe landing and prayers offered for help with my enterprise. My request, however, was ambivalent. As a supplicant I found myself in the unusual position of wishing to be successful, but not too much so; of wanting to present myself in the best possible light to the institutions I would be visiting, but not to the point where I would be given serious consideration. I had no desire to go to medical school – anywhere. The best possible result for me? To have a good time and at the end of the trip be able to truthfully say to Bertha that I had made a sincere effort, gave it my best shot, but for whatever reason (e.g., too late in the application process), I was unsuccessful. Then, finally, I could get on with my career in the Air Force. I was using my own money throughout, so my conscience would be clear in that regard.

The train from Limerick to Cork initially followed what I assumed to be the Shannon River, along which were closely spaced farms. Their stonewalled fields were riddled with gray rock around which gaunt cattle nibbled the brown-green sod. We passed a series of dry swamps, their sides sharply cut, with stacks of earth piled nearby. I later learned these were peat bogs and when the wedges of turf dried out, they were used as fuel. Workers in the fields waved as we passed.

In my coach there was a group of about twelve young men heading to a sports event in Cork. They were in great spirits, heightened perhaps by accompanying libations. Soon a small accordion appeared and then a penny flute. The music, singing, and drinking, continued for the duration of the journey. I didn't recognize any of their offerings but assumed they were rebel songs or related to their team and county. The whole scene was almost a caricature of what one would expect in a John Ford-directed Irish movie. All that was missing was Barry Fitzgerald walking through collecting tickets. It was all great fun, and I decided that later in the evening I would try some of that black beer everyone was drinking.

Upon arrival in Cork, I chanced upon the Metropole Hotel, ideally located in the center of the city. The room was small but very clean. After dinner I struck up a conversation with the receptionist – small talk about the city, her job, and where she went to school.

"I go to the University of Cork," she said. "I love it...And have you ever been to Cork before?"

"No, first time," I said.

"Then let me take you up on the roof. It's not busy and the view is smashing."

And so it was. At that time, the hotel was one of the taller buildings in Cork, and the perimeter of the city was clearly visible. In the distance the River Lee, making its way to the sea, shimmered in the glow of early evening. The receptionist spoke of her interest in America, explaining that she had relatives there whom she hoped to visit one day. She was cute – auburn hair with clear white skin dotted with freckles - but her accent was anything but lilting. I thanked her for the "tour." That night, I slept the sleep of the very weary, my money and passport tucked safely under my pillow.

A Day at the Beach

The following day, Monday, was a bank holiday; everything, including the college, was closed. I inquired at the desk whether they had any suggestions on how to spend the day. The consensus was a bus trip to Crosshaven, a popular beach destination which drew large crowds. It sounded like a fun thing to do, and I would get to see some of the local area.

At the terminal I boarded the assigned bus, luckily found a seat, and headed off on a beautiful Irish morning. I was aware of looks in my direction. Americans were not as ubiquitous as they are today, more of a rare species worthy of a sideward glance. My seatmate, a rotund, older gentleman wearing glasses, initiated conversation.

"So where do you live in the U.S.?"

"Rhode Island," I answered, and assuming that he'd never heard of our tiny state, added, "It's located between--"

"Ah sure, I know it well," he interrupted. "Lived in the states a number of years and saw much of the country. Had a wonderful time. Then, surely, you must be a sailor. I've been to Newport, beautiful place."

"I live across the bay but so far haven't sailed, maybe someday."

We chatted on and I soon learned he was something of a history buff. With little prodding he shared some of the lore connected to our destination. Sir Francis Drake had sought cover in Crosshaven when chased by the Spanish Armada in the 1500s, and the distress messages from the torpedoed Lusitania, in 1915, were first picked up there. Roger Casement was captured, just up the coast, attempting to smuggle arms to the rebels during the 1916 uprising against the British. Additionally, across the bay was Cobh, the Ireland terminus for transatlantic liners, and incidentally, the last port visited by the Titanic.

At one of our longer stops, he invited me for a drink as a small payback. He seemed pretty straight so we went to a nearby pub and had what I believe was a John Jameson and lime - a nice gesture.

The bus deposited us in front of a series of small shops which catered to the needs of the day-tripping beachgoer. Just beyond, a path through a wooded area led to a gate, which for a fee of six-pence, allowed entrance. A steep incline led to a narrow and extremely rocky shore, along which groups of people were scattered. Flat stretches along the face of the hill served as picnic sites for families. Those swimming were mostly young people, some wearing scapulas. Other than face and forearms, no one had a tan. Taking off my shoes, I walked the beach, the sand gritty and scattered with stones and shells, the water freezing.

In the late afternoon the buses lined up for the trip back to the city. I found a seat in one, crowded with bodies hot and sweaty after the long day, faces flushed with sunburn, babies crying, and pungent with the smell of oranges and cigarettes. Murmurs of conversation became muted as we made our way through small villages en route to the city. Then a chorus of whoops broke out when we pulled into Cork.

The next morning I visited the University of Cork: a pleasant campus with Tudor Gothic buildings ringing a central quadrangle and well-groomed grounds enclosed by a massive iron fence. The lady at the admissions office was helpful and encouraged me to fill out the application papers. But when I asked about the chance of joining this year's class, she offered a rueful smile.

"No, you'll have no chance this year." Then she added, "Even if someone drops out, there's a list of those waiting to take that place."

I thanked her for her time. While not exactly welcomed with open arms, I had at least officially started the process which was the purpose of my trip.

That night I had a couple of beers at the hotel bar. As I was finishing a visit to the men's room, a man walked in standing well over six feet tall, with a girth to match. He was well turned out in a suit and tie, quite handsome, with a full head of black hair, combed straight back: an imposing figure.

Later, I noticed him at the center of a group of people. When he left, I asked the barman, "Who was he?"

"Jack Doyle, a boxer, fought for the British Heavyweight Championship once."

"Never heard of him," I replied.

The barman said, "That's not surprising; he never trained, so never won very much but did get to that level. In those days, he looked like a bloody movie star; women flocked to Doyle. To cap it all he had a voice that was compared to John McCormick's." He paused and smiled. "A few years later when he could barely last a couple rounds, the craic (joke) was - he boxed like John McCormick and sang like Jack Dempsey.

"Doyle married a woman named Movita, a Hollywood actress," the barman continued. "The story goes, she left Howard Hughes for Jack. They used to come into the bar whenever they were in town. But I guess they got fighting. Jack liked his "drop," and I think he popped her a couple of times. Movita used to complain to me that Jack drank too much. Although I sympathized with her, I also told her, 'That's what you get when you marry an Irishman.'" The barman excused himself and went off to serve another customer.

You should meet my family, the people who brought me up, I thought. *One hundred percent Irish and totally abstinent.* Aunt Bertha once confided that her mother confessed to her the reason she'd married her dad was not only because he was Catholic, but as important, he didn't drink. Knowing my grandmother, I wasn't totally surprised, but I would like to think there was a jigger or two of affection in the mix.

And myself, soon to be out in the world on my own, freed from the constraints of college and family, might I not develop a "thirst" and be inexorably drawn by some anomalous chromosome to the drink – the dark side of my heritage? Would I one day be sprawled in some hole of a bar, babbling to a chalk-faced harpy of my time in the sun, of the good life I'd let slip through my fingers? Who knew what lay ahead? Unsettled by the possibility, I signaled the barman for another stout.

As he served my drink, I asked, "What's Jack doing these days?"

"Well," he replied, "Movita eventually divorced him and married Marlon Brando. And it was pretty much downhill for Jack after that, although he's still looking good...you saw him. I hear he's living in England. He sings in a couple of clubs and someone said he's taken up wrestling."

Years later I heard that Jack had become a down and out drunk, living off a small stipend from his divorce; eventually he died from cirrhosis of the liver at age 65. Another instance of an Irishman with a ton of talent who, to paraphrase the singer, Christy Moore, laments in *The Contender:*

> "...was born beneath a star that promised all,
> who could have lived his life between Cork, Cobh, and Youghal,
> but the wheel of fortune took him
> and from the highest point it shook him,
> by the bottle live, by the bottle he did fall."

The following morning, I took the train to Dublin, arriving at Kingsbridge Station in the late afternoon. A bed and breakfast was found near Phoenix Park - the largest park in Ireland. It was comprised of about 3,800 acres of playing fields, nature trails, animal enclosures, and bicycle paths: an oasis in a teeming industrial city.

Tea that evening was shared with an English couple touring Ireland. The friendliness and rapport between them and the Irish landlady amazed me; I had presumed an animosity as a part of their respective DNA. Although I'm aware that there are business aspects to consider when running a guest house, including treating the guests well, the sociability seemed genuine. My status as an American provoked much discussion, everyone curious as to how life "really" was in the United States. They asked questions relating to politics and entertainment: "Do you think this Kennedy chap has a chance at President?" "Have you ever seen Frank Sinatra?" "Have you ever been to Las Vegas?" I tried to answer a host of queries with a minimum of fabrication.

The discussions were friendly and the majority of the comments complimentary to the United States. Although delighted with their opinion of the States, I made an effort not to come across as the "ugly American" who decrees that "everything's bigger and better in the good ol' U.S. of A."

"The American tourists that come to the British Isles and Ireland each year," I insisted, "are here because you guys have something that we don't – so it all evens out. But visit us one day and see what you think."

They all agreed they'd love to.

The Quest Continues

The next day, armed with copies of my diploma and transcripts of my grades, I visited the medical schools in Ireland's largest city. University College Dublin was my first stop, and although I had been told by the professor before my trip that the 1955 class was filled, I still put in an application. The clerk at the registrar's office was not very optimistic, even for 1956.

Likewise, Trinity College was no exception. Applications to their medical school were sent to an address in England. I took the required information, but the gentleman I spoke with offered little hope.

The impressive facade of the College, however, invited exploration. The arched entrance of the gatehouse was attended by a well-attired man of apparent authority who, after inquiring as to my business, permitted entrance. Just beyond, a cobblestoned courtyard was dignified by a ring of imposing Doric-columned gray stone buildings. Formerly an Augustinian monastery, the buildings were converted to a college during the reign of Queen Elizabeth I, in order to provide a "proper education" for the sons and daughters of the English occupiers. The Book of Kells, a legacy of the monks of Iona, was housed in the library.

Past the quadrangle were the playing fields - a broad sweep of green encircled by a running track. The day I visited, a cricket match was in progress. A few spectators stretched out on the grass or leisurely strolled about, with seemingly, a very relaxed involvement in the match. Even the occasional applause seemed restrained, creating an atmosphere which I took to be quintessentially British.

Leaving Trinity, I crossed the street to the American Express office. It had been arranged that Aunt Bertha would be in touch via letters to American Express, in whichever major city she thought I would be at the time. I was not surprised to find a letter from her in their office. She expressed her usual admonitions to eat plenty of salads and fruit, not to lose my money, and to be especially careful of my passport. The last paragraph looked like this:

...I had a conversation with a gentleman I met at a lecture. His son recently received a medical degree from the Royal College of Physicians and Surgeons in Dublin. He's now practicing in Canada. So, Gene, if he was accepted in Canada, the degree probably would be good in the U.S. So be sure to apply there when you're in Dublin!

I was beginning to wonder if Bertha discussed anything else on her trip besides her medical school search agenda.

The American Express office was located at the bottom of Grafton Street and I was told that the College of Surgeons was located at the opposite end. The walk to the College took me up a busy thoroughfare lined with shops and department stores, crowded with people, unrushed, enjoying the warmth of the day. Knots of by-standers chatted on narrow sidewalks. Vehicles inched their way along the bustling street, drivers honked their impatience, a violinist performed while a young boy by his side held out a cap. On I walked; a marvelous aroma vented from a coffee shop, an old woman begged for coins by a church lane, and then came the breakout at the top of the street. I was informed that the unremarkable gray building just up the block was the Royal College of Surgeons.

"No," was the curt reply I received from a heavyset woman with ink-stained fingers in the registrar's office, when I asked for an application. "Classes are set for the coming year," she informed me. When I persisted and asked if I could at least have an application on file at the College, she turned without answer-

41

ing and went back to a paper-strewn desk at the far end of the room. With further conversation unlikely, I left the building and crossed the street to a large park, later identified as St. Stephens Green.

The longer I walked around the manicured, flower-filled gardens of the Green, the more annoyed I became at the rude dismissal, the first instance of that in Ireland. The notion of rejection, to which I was becoming accustomed, didn't grate as much as the woman's attitude. There wasn't any reason, I felt, why I couldn't at least get my name in the mix. Frustrated, I turned and headed back to the college.

A different woman, younger than the previous one, stood behind the counter. Patiently, she listened to my tale and affirmed that they were instructed not to give out applications when classes were filled for the year. Would it be possible, I wondered aloud, to write a short note to the registrar, indicating my interest? My plea was buttressed with an indication of the distance traveled and the unlikelihood of my having this opportunity again.

The young lady smiled, agreed that it was a bit irregular, but probably wouldn't do any harm. Provided with a sheet of paper and pen, I composed a note which briefly outlined my background and provided contact information. With tongue in cheek, I also indicated a sincere desire to become a physician.

A copy of my college transcript and diploma, along with the note and five pounds (the application fee), were sealed in a manila envelope, addressed to the registrar and placed, with similar envelopes, on a side table.

I leaned over the counter and shook the woman's hand. "I really appreciate the help. You didn't have to do any of this."

"Hope it works out."

"Do you smoke?" I asked.

She nodded. I gave her my unopened pack of Lucky Strikes.

"Thanks very much. I've never smoked American cigarettes

before." She hesitated for a moment, then reached over to the side table and retrieved my envelope. "I'll personally see that this is on the registrar's desk in the morning."

In those days, American cigarettes and dollar bills were a currency unto themselves.

The B & I Adventure

That night I planned to depart Ireland for Liverpool via the B&I Steamship Line. After a two-decker bus dropped me at the O'Connell Street Bridge, I made my way along the quays to the ship. Across the river, windows blazed in a late afternoon sun and on this luminous evening, even the dirty, debris-ridden Liffey River had a turgid appeal.

At dockside, hundreds of people waited to board. Local pubs bustled with business. Most of the passengers, home for the bank holiday, were returning to their jobs in England. Many young men were dressed in the mod Teddy Boy fashion, a throwback to the day of the Edwardian dandy: long jackets, drain pipe pants, open white shirts with shoestring ties, and hair slicked back into DA's (ducks' asses). Uniform in tight sweaters, toreador pants, and high heels, the young women smoked cigarettes and looked fashionably bored.

The gangplank lowered and the rush was on for choice spots in the lounges. As it was such a beautiful evening, I decided to stay on deck with the hope that a good looking female would wish to share the sunset with me. Past cranes and cargo ships, we made our way down a placid Liffey and once past the breakwater lights at the harbor entrance, felt the first tremors of the Irish Sea. A fellow passenger identified Howth Head and the smudge of Killiney in the distance.

A cold, wet wind cleared the deck. Below, all seats and much of the deck floor were taken. I promptly found and appropriated a space against the curved hull. Through the night, the ship creaked and strained as it rolled through heavy seas; a thickening fog of cigarette smoke settled over the room as did an overpowering smell of bodies. There were only snatches of sleep. A girl in black stockings, seated opposite, grew more attractive as the night plodded along. Later, with the sea rougher, Miss Black

Stockings, along with others, became sick, and my interest suddenly cooled. The stench was so strong it could be tasted. This was how it must have been for those on the immigrant ships to America: almost unbearable.

Some hours later there was a change in the engine pitch. Curious, I went on deck; the night was clear, the water calm. In the distance winked the lights of England. Being young and sporting an Irish sentimentality, this indeed was a momentous occasion.

As we approached Liverpool's port, the ship passed through a seemingly endless series of locks. Since everything was still new and exciting, I remained on deck, watching the locks open and close until about 7:00 a.m., when we reached the harbor. A British naval officer, returning home after a long period at sea, pointed out the Royal Liver Building with its foreboding lions, gargoyle-like, perched at its corners. This was, for many seamen headed into the North Sea during WW II, their last sight of England. The dreary, misty morning was an apt introduction to a dull, gray city.

As we disembarked I noticed that my black-stockinged friend was met by a mustached Teddy boy type, who didn't seem overly happy to be there.

My sailor acquaintance had recommended a bed & breakfast where he had stayed. Fortunately, rooms were available, and soon I was enjoying a breakfast of eggs, rasher (bacon), and toast. After the meal I stretched out on the bed, fell asleep, and stayed there most of the day.

Surfacing in late afternoon, my mood was as foul as the weather. *What in the hell was I doing in this miserable city, in this crummy B&B, on this ridiculous fool's errand?* I thought of chucking the whole project and going home. Later that evening I explored a foggy and dismal Liverpool and eventually went to a movie, *The Dam Busters*, which starred Richard Todd. Interestingly, smoking was allowed in the theater.

After I checked out of the B&B the following morning, I took a bus to the University of Liverpool. Other than the accent, there was no change in the message. Even if space had been available, which it wasn't, an English Leaving Certificate equivalent and three letters of recommendation from practicing English physicians were required before consideration. The final comment from the clerk was, "You'd better go home, Yank," accompanied by a sarcastic laugh.

Not in a good mood to start, my immediate thought was to respond along the lines of, "Listen, you sonofabitch, you wouldn't have your stupid little job if the Yanks hadn't rescued your miserable little country, you asshole."

"Thank you for your time," were the words that came out of my mouth and I moved on.

The plan was to go to London after Liverpool but while waiting for a ticket booth to open at the station, I noticed a train scheduled for Edinburgh, leaving within the hour. "Why not give it a shot?" The University in Edinburgh had a medical school and anything was more appealing than what I had encountered so far in England. Also, Aunt Bertha would be traveling through Edinburgh in the next few days; maybe we could arrange a reunion.

The train was a typical English carriage: compartments, entered through sliding glass doors, with facing seats for three to four passengers on either side. Racks for luggage were above each seat. Shortly after leaving Liverpool, the weather improved. The sun appeared and my sour mood of the previous day quickly dissipated.

Within an hour the grayness of the bleak city was replaced by a verdant countryside. Vistas of green fields stretched in all directions, interrupted occasionally by tracts of woodland and small villages. Heightened by a brilliant morning sun, a kaleidoscope of images - small farms, cattle grazing, distant hills, and bicyclists on narrow roads - flowed by the windows. At stops along the way, stations were attractively decorated with flower gardens and window boxes.

A minister and his wife and daughter were my compartment companions. Returning from holidays, they were headed home to a small village south of Edinburgh. Pleasant conversation was shared which included anything I could tell them of America. Their daughter and I shared a fleeting glance or two, which I felt boded well. An invitation was extended to visit if I were ever in their area. They took the time to write their address so I assumed the offer was sincere. But alas, I never did visit their little village or find out if it's true what's said about minister's daughters.

The train station in Edinburgh was adjacent to the Royal Caledonian Hotel, where Bertha's group would be staying. Their visit coincided with the Edinburgh Festival, a celebrated annual event, which attracted large crowds from the British Isles, Europe, and the United States. As a result, accommodations of any kind were at a premium. My search began along Princess Street, Edinburgh's broad main thoroughfare, filled this day with hundreds of people strolling and browsing the shops. In the distance, perched on massive volcanic rock, stood Edinburgh Castle, the wide swath of green at its base speckled with people enjoying a balmy late afternoon.

Over the next several hours, attempts to secure lodging were not successful. Soon I found myself a good distance from the city center, well into the residential area of Edinburgh. The long twilight gave the impression of a lingering late afternoon, but now, around ten o'clock, the night was fast approaching and my pursuit acquired a hint of desperation. A small park provided a place to stop and assess the situation. I decided to leave my bag behind some bushes and thus, unencumbered, move more quickly. If a place were found I'd retrieve the bag. If not, I'd sleep in the park. The night was mild without a hint of rain.

A short distance from the green, I came to yet another bed and breakfast. The usual reply was expected and I was not disappointed. The oft-repeated tale of my lengthy search made little impression on the landlady. "Just for tonight," I implored. "I'll take anything you have."

The lady hesitated; I sensed a flicker of hope. She said she would talk to her husband, with whom she returned a few minutes later. A short, stalwart chap, he looked me up and down, said nothing and left. The lady indicated there was a room in the cellar portion of the house where I could stay temporarily. "It's the maid's room," she added. "She's on vacation and is due back in two days. Would that be alright?" Too choked up to answer I nodded yes.

After retrieving my bag, I returned and was shown a small bed in a small room. A grander suite I could not have imagined.

"I hope," the landlady said, "that you enjoy your stay with us." (Neither she nor I could have imagined the ground-breaking events which would play out during my short time there.) "Come upstairs to the dining room after you unpack."

Following her instructions I found a small supper for me,

a very nice gesture. After a bath, I crawled between two clean sheets, totally exhausted. My last recollection was the song "Cherry Pink and Apple Blossom White" being played in the adjoining room.

Breakfast the following morning was the British staple of rasher, eggs, toast in a rack, and a small dish of butter balls surrounded by chips of ice. My fellow diners didn't have the taut tourist look − or a map tilted against the salt and pepper shakers - more the relaxed bearing of boarders. Seated by the window was an attractive blonde, sipping a cup of tea and smoking a cigarette. When leaving the room she passed by my table, offered a nod, and the hint of a smile.

In the light of day it was apparent that my room was quite removed from the main house, with a separate entrance from the street. A single window looked onto a patch of green in the back yard. The only other room in the basement was the one adjacent, presumably the source of last night's serenade. Seeking out the landlady I again expressed my appreciation, then headed out on a gorgeous morning to explore the city.

On my return, early afternoon, the door to the adjoining room was ajar. The blonde woman whom I had seen at breakfast appeared. Music was playing in the background.

"Hello there; I just want to apologize for the racket last night. Thought Ann had come back early from vacation. Hope I didn't disturb you." Her accent was foreign, probably French. "And, by the way, I'm Maria."

"Nice to meet you; I'm Gene." We shook hands. "Don't be sorry. A brass band wouldn't have bothered me last night. Good song, though; Herb Alpert, right?"

She nodded yes. "I love his music," she said. Tall with nice eyes and a good figure, Maria appeared to be in her mid-twenties. A quick glance revealed no rings.

"I was about to make myself a drink, Gene, something cool for this warm afternoon. If you've nothing planned, why don't you join me? I'll make amends for last night and you can tell me what's brought you to Edinburgh."

I nodded. "Sounds good."

Her room, although larger, was otherwise similar to mine. A light perfume scent was evident. After clothes were cleared, I sat in the only chair; Maria sat on the side of the bed. The conversation was mainly introductory. Maria was Austrian, born in Vienna, and schooled in France. A modeling contract had brought her to Edinburgh, and when finished in the fall, she'd return to Paris.

"Edinburgh's a nice city," she added, "but it's not Paris. I can't wait to get back."

Briefly, I described my background and medical school quest. "My plan is to go to Paris after London, mainly to see the city; I can't imagine any medical school possibilities there."

"Don't be too sure, Gene. The Sorbonne's a great school, especially in medicine. A lot of foreigners go there."

Drinking gin and tonics in the middle of an afternoon with an attractive woman who had a French accent, and seemed to like me, was a situation with which I was not familiar. She asked if there was a girlfriend at home. After my negative response, she commented that she couldn't believe that such a nice-looking man (not boy) didn't have *many*. The compliment, though brushed off, was reveled in.

The conversation, increasingly more relaxed, continued: a recent birthday celebrated her twenty-sixth year; marriage, which had been "endured" for four years, ended in divorce. No children resulted, and although not discussed, she alluded to an inability to have any. Things were becoming hazy but pleasantly so.

"Do you like French music?" she asked abruptly.

At this point I liked everything. "Don't know much about it," I answered. "But, I like music, no matter where it's from; I just like music. If it's good, it's good." Profound statements such as these I always found more available after a few drinks.

"Well," she said, "I have a favorite, which I'm sure you'll like."

The record was *Cabaret Night in Paris* and although I did not know it at the time, it was to become our anthem. We played it constantly. The songs included Charles Trenet's "La Mer," "J'Attendrai" with Tino Rossi, Edith Piaf's "La Vie En Rose," along with Jean Sablon and others, all sung in the French cabaret tradition. Listening led to dancing. Dancing led to kissing. Kissing led to touching and along the way we drank the remaining gin.

At this juncture it might be appropriate to place this situation in the context of me at age twenty-one. I was a product of a rigid, religious, Irish-Catholic home where terms of endearment were avoided, and the dictates of the bishop and Baltimore Catechism strictly applied. Sex was never a word, let alone a topic, mentioned in our house. Christian Brothers in high school were followed by Jesuits in college. Holy Cross was all male at that time. Mass was compulsory five times a week, Sunday being optional. If you missed two of the five services, you were "campused" for the following weekend (which required punching a clock every three hours to ensure you didn't stray far). Freshman year we had 10 p.m. bed checks, with curfews for the remaining three years (except on weekends). No women or alcohol were allowed in the residencies - a disciplinary package as strict as the service academies, it was said. The highlight of the year was the annual retreat where a fire-and-brimstone Retreat Master would outline in some detail, the things one shouldn't do with the opposite sex. For many of us, the revelations of the sins we were admonished to avoid only whetted an appetite for their commission.

The extent of my social and sexual interactions comprised a few kisses and the occasional backseat wrestle. My work-related aroma during the summers effectively negated any consensual activity. My virginity was intact. Suffice to say, one could not have been more naive than I was that summer of 1955 in Edinburgh, Scotland.

Maria eventually suggested food, and since it was such a beautiful day, she thought it would be fun to have a late picnic. After we picked up sandwiches at a local shop we headed to the same green I utilized the previous night. Stretched out on a blanket, my companion sunbathed in the waning light and in the process displayed a terrific figure. Conversation moved easily, during which she mentioned a recent break-up with a boyfriend. Apparently, after she left Paris, he found a greener pasture.

On the way home we stopped to visit Elspeth, a friend of Maria's and a fellow model. Elspeth, a native of Scotland, was tall, very attractive, but painfully thin. She was planning a party at her place later that evening and said she'd be delighted if we both came by. The invitation was accepted.

Maria was able to schedule a hair appointment that evening which gave me a chance for a quick nap and an opportunity to get some clothes washed. My wardrobe was quite limited but the landlady kindly ironed my last clean, but wrinkled, shirt. Restored by the nap, I was set for the night.

Many artsy types, friends of Elspeth's from her school days, were in attendance. Maria and I spent most of the evening dancing and drinking. At the end of the night, accompanied by a pleasant glow, we found our way home.

Back in her room, Maria put on our record. When I approached her to dance, she backed away. "Give me a moment, Gene," she said. I sat on the side of the bed and watched her.

Inclining her head, she removed her earrings, then her beaded necklace, placing them carefully in a jewelry box on the dresser. Once loosened from its braid and shaken free, her blond hair cascaded down her back. Leaning against the only chair in the room, she kicked off her shoes.

Coming towards me she undid the top button of her dress, which after a shrug of her shoulders, fell in a shimmer of light to the floor.

There I sat, beholding what I had seen only fleetingly before and wanting to do what I'd never done before, yet feeling so self-righteous and morally superior. All that had been pumped into me over the years filled my brain as I looked upon this "wanton woman."

Her gaze was direct, her smile coy. "Perhaps, mon cher," she said, her voice a smokey whisper, "you could help with the rest."

This was the precise moment I'd been warned of: the particular circumstance when moral Catholic youth are meant to cobble together a flurry of Hail Mary's, which when rendered with conviction and fervor, would quell the surge of unwholesome thoughts.

At that point, remembering my middle name was a challenge, let alone a Hail Mary. Nor had I any interest in stifling my desire. But I did recollect, in the nick of time, that most accommodating of Sacraments: Confession. The assurance of eventual absolution cleared my mind. When Maria reached for me, a pressure too long deferred, became insistent, and so it was, with some urgency, that I took her hands and drew her to me.

If I walked with something of a bounce in my step the following morning, a Sunday, I felt it was warranted. Critiquing my performance, I thought I had done fairly well, an opinion that Maria shared on at least two occasions. Although fireworks were not noted at the climactic moment, the attendant shortness of breath did induce a pleasant hypoxia. Maria was still sleeping when I left, and in spite of what had occurred the previous night, or perhaps because of it, I found a Catholic church and went to Mass. The guilt that I presumed would weigh heavily, failed to surface. Communion, however, was not taken, in recognition of my transgression.

After Mass I explored Edinburgh, and when I returned in the early afternoon, there was a note from Maria saying she had gone to the beach with some friends.

> So sorry I missed you this morning. Went swimming, wished you could come, on it is a party. Shirt is in the wardrobe. Do phone me, Terrible sorry you have to move. Hope you got fixed up allright.
>
> love
>
> Maria.
>
> CEN 4344
>
> Giles please!

As the maid would soon be returning, I needed to find another place to stay. Miraculously, lodging was found on Dublin Street, about two blocks away. Later, Maria and I went to dinner, enjoyed some dancing, then - back to her room.

The following day, at the University of Edinburgh, the standard response remained intact. Classes were full for the year. Nevertheless I did put in an application, followed by a tour of Edinburgh Castle. When I inquired at the Royal Caledonian, I was told that Bertha's group was not expected for another three days. I decided to go to London, try the schools there, then return and meet my aunt.

Maria saw me off with a return promised in a few days. In London, a room was found, shared with three others, in a seedy establishment near the King's Cross train station. Rooming houses near stations, although handy for the traveler, were suspect in the areas of security and cleanliness, and at first glance, this place maintained that perception.

Walking about the city that afternoon, quite by chance, I came upon many of London's tourist attractions: 10 Downing Street, Westminster Abbey, and Berkeley Square, absent the nightingale. Much of the evening was spent in and around Piccadilly Circus, a hub of activity somewhat similar to New York's Times Square. The diversity of nationalities, the parade of styles, and the unfamiliar accents seemed so European, so cosmopolitan.

I located two medical schools the following day: Kings College and the institution affiliated with Barts Hospital. Considerable time, in both instances, was spent finding the right building, the right office in the building, and the right person in the office - the one who dealt with medical school admissions. The final links were similarly pleasant, blank-faced ladies, equally unfamiliar with admission procedures as they were processed at different locations. They supplied me with those addresses.

That particular day epitomized the futility of my quixotic quest. Perhaps London intimidated me, with its crowds, traffic, cavernous buildings - the bustle and impersonality of a large city. But, almost as an epiphany, I recognized the whole endeavor for what it was: tedious, dispiriting and unrealistic - a waste of time. When I met Aunt Bertha in a day or two, I'd convince her of the ridiculousness of her improbable notion, insist it was time to ring the curtain down, and head home. The only pleasant distraction on that dismal day was the thought of Maria and her supple body.

Back in Edinburgh, I reclaimed my digs on Dublin Street. Later I met Maria, and we headed to the neighborhood bar, a dimly lit room in the basement portion of a townhouse. After a couple of "our" drinks (Gordon's Gin and Schweppes tonic), and a small supper, we went back to her place. Charles Trenet, Edith Piaf and the others were waiting. It was a fine night.

A call to the Royal Caledonian Hotel the following morning informed me that Aunt Bertha was out on a tour but they were expected back about three o'clock in the afternoon.

"Had a little tie-up in traffic," the receptionist told me when I asked at the desk about Bertha's group. "Probably be another thirty or so minutes. There's a comfortable lounge," she said, nodding toward the front of the hotel. "You'll be able to see them when they pull in."

Sauntering over, I sank into the sofa, put my feet up on the footstool and stretched out. Across the room, sitting at a round table scattered with magazines, was an older woman and a young boy who was writing in what appeared to be a notebook. The woman intently watched his efforts.

Now there's a flashback. Countless hours had been spent with Bertha at such a table from elementary through high school. Reviewing my homework, helping with a composition, answering questions on quizzes she devised, was a daily ritual. Bertha's focus on education was intense and unrelenting.

She had never married, but even her choice of boyfriends included a learning component for me. Matt Flynn, a classics professor at Providence College, gave me weekly tutorials in Latin while he and Bertha were an item; Fritz Statler (who drove a neat little coupe with a rumble-seat), took me flying in his open cockpit, bi-plane. Basic flight instruction was shouted from

Fritz in the rear seat. Mal Williams, a track coach at the University of Rhode Island, was coerced by Bertha into providing running technique and training. An insurance agent, Frank Mason instructed me in the essentials of his business. My relations with all of her male friends were fraught with anxiety, worrying that one might marry her and then she would leave me. But that never happened.

When the lady across the lounge left, presumably to go to the ladies room, the young boy stopped writing and began reading one of the magazines on the table. When he saw the woman reappear, he pushed it away quickly. Preparing to leave, she put her arm around the boy's shoulder and gave him a hug. He looked up at her and smiled back. It looked like a happy smile.

Sure enough, I had a clear view of the large tourist bus when it pulled up across the street to disgorge Bertha's party, about 25 women. Taller than the others, red hair wind-blown, Aunt Bertha was not to be missed. Carriage erect, she had the gait of an athlete, a legacy of her years as a physical education teacher. Her strong, angular facial features frequently brought comparison to Katherine Hepburn. In 1955 Bertha was forty-eight years old but any woman ten years younger would be complimented by the comparison.

Pleased and surprised to see me, we went off for a cup of tea. Intently, she listened to all that had transpired since my arrival in Ireland. Positive at the outset, I eventually admitted discouragement. Throughout the conversation, in various guises, I implied that any thought of a positive outcome was unrealistic. She wasn't too upset with the lack of progress and reminded me of the fall-back plan that had been agreed upon - to go to France and the Continent - if things didn't work out here. I nodded that I remembered.

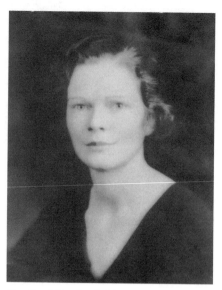

Bertha Elizabeth McKee 1907-2008

"Anyway...," I hesitated, "I've given it a lot of thought, Bertha; I think it's time to throw in the towel and go home."

"Oh, really?" Bertha replied. She quickly drank her tea. "And what, may I ask, are you going to do when you get there?"

"Get my job back, I suppose, until it's time to head to Texas."

"So you'd rather cut fish than go to Paris. Is that what I'm hearing?"

"Well, no, Bertha, you don't understand..."

Bertha was becoming agitated, never a good sign. "Of course I understand," she fired back. "You've decided to pass up an opportunity that you may never have again so you can work in a fish factory for a couple of weeks. Of course, I understand; I especially understand stupidity."

"It's a waste of time, Bertha."

"So's cutting fish, and so's the Air Force, as far as I'm concerned." She called to the waitress for another cup of tea. "Look, you've come this far. You simply can't quit now; if nothing else, do it for the experience."

"It's a waste of money," I countered, appealing to her frugal side.

"Do you have enough for two or three weeks?" Her tea was being stirred vigorously.

I shrugged my shoulders. "Probably, but it's hard to tell."

"You'll never forgive yourself if you quit now, you know."

I sat in silence. *I already have*, I thought.

"Well?" she asked.

"Anyway, how about the language?" I asked. "I can't speak French if you haven't noticed."

"You can learn it."

I realized I wasn't going to win this battle.

"Well?" she asked again.

"OK, Bertha; I guess I can hang in for a couple of weeks."

"Have you made any arrangements for Paris yet?"

"No, I wanted to talk to you first."

"Well, you'd better get going on it."

With the decision made, Bertha was more relaxed. Her trip was going well; the group got along famously, and she was looking forward to the rest of the itinerary, which included Ireland. Their flight home would be out of Shannon.

I was tempted to tell Bertha about Maria but decided against it. Her response would be predictable: "You're not over here to chase women." Secondly, my discussion of women with Bertha was such a rare topic, the antennae would immediately go up – questions would begin and a lecture would soon follow. My desire to tell the world of my first conquest would have to wait.

Unfortunately, the conversation soon returned to the "project" as Bertha called it. Various positive scenarios were discussed. While Bertha arranged my future, the only thought in my head was how I could politely work a "Good night" into the conversation and get back to Maria.

The teachers left two days later; I saw them off. Bertha wanted to take my picture and in a fit of adolescent pique I refused, and she felt badly. We settled for one of our infrequent hugs. The envelope she handed me, after the second hug, contained forty-five dollars.

Over drinks that evening I told Maria of my plans for Paris and of my departure within the next day or so. The remaining time we had was spent in her room drinking gin and tonics, smoking Senior Service cigarettes, and having sex, interrupted only by the occasional deli run. We were never drunk but always high, never so weary of sex that we didn't want more, and never so tired of Tino and the cabaret crew that we considered listening to anyone else. There was nothing specific to remember of those days: only a blur of time when no thought went unspoken and no sensation was left unexplored.

In conversation with my landlady, I mentioned my Paris destination, and my lack of a place to stay. A priest, she recalled, had stayed with her a year or two earlier, who lived outside Paris and who, she believed, took in boarders. Going through her records she found his name and address. So, with a bit of serendipity, I had the address of Father Montgomery Wright, 30 Avenue de Longchamps, Val d'Or, France.

Maria saw me off, tearful and clinging. She promised to write. Looking at her as we said our goodbyes, I was mystified at how this strikingly attractive woman had developed a fancy for me. But ours, it is said, is not to reason why... and certainly not to complain.

Purchase at Petticoat Lane

In London I found a room near the Euston train station which I shared with three others: two teenagers on holiday and an out-of-work musician. As before, it was a wallet and passport-under-the-pillow type of establishment.

The following day, August 15th, the Assumption of the Blessed Virgin Mary, I went to Mass. (Looking back at that time in my life, I'm amazed at how inculcated I was in things Catholic. Now, the Holy Days pass without a thought, unless reminded.)

After Mass, with a free afternoon until my departure that night, I acted on a suggestion from my musician roommate and visited Petticoat Lane. The original center of London's clothing market, hence its name, was a large outdoor market with hundreds of tents, booths, wagons, and stalls, which sold just about anything imaginable. Strolling musicians and small bands added entertainment.

Vendors circulated in the crowd hawking their goods. One was selling little wooden boxes with two rollers attached that could be turned with a small metal crank, like an old-fashioned clothes dryer. The man, with frequent glances over his shoulder, inserted a piece of white paper into one side of the roller, turned the crank and a pound note emerged from the other side. After every sale the fellow would hurry off to another spot. In a conspiratorial tone he explained to the three or four of us that followed him, "It's the coppers (police). The locals (stores) are losing a few quid and they've got the hounds out. It's the poor I'm trying to help, Matey. And the bastards won't leave me alone."

He claimed to have only a half dozen boxes left, and when they were sold he was going into hiding in Europe. He allowed me to buy one - the sale including a sheaf of thin, white papers - before he disappeared into the crowd again. I never figured out why, in spite of doing everything exactly as demonstrated, I was never able to produce a pound note.

Later that afternoon I entrained to Dover and then boarded the ferry to Dieppe. Compared to the B&I ship out of Dublin, this was a luxury liner. Easing our way through a crowded harbor, the ship's passengers soon enjoyed a beautiful evening on the English Channel. Off in the distance were Dover's limestone cliffs, reviving memories of Vera Lynn and bomber pilots returning from Europe who welcomed the landmark signifying home. We passed through the waters where once swept the D-Day flotilla and where Spitfires in the skies overhead fought the Battle of Britain; all I had heard and read about, now vicariously shared. I thought it was really neat.

As the gray night stealthily approached, on we plowed through the choppy seas towards France, my first truly foreign country. The thought brought a sudden shudder, a sensation familiar from other times when I had to face the unknown. Alone on deck, I found a small space behind a protruding metal strut, wide enough for me to sit and be out of the wind.

Huddled in my cave, landfall in Dieppe hours away, my mind churned with questions, each more unanswerable than the last. *How will I find my way when I arrive in Paris if I can't ask for directions? If I'm lost, who do I call for help? How will I buy a ticket or change money or read train schedules?* The only connection I had with a human being in France was a name and address written on a small piece of paper in my wallet. *Will I be able to find the town where the priest lives? What if he's moved? Then what will I do? Do I have enough money to survive?*

One after the other, the thoughts cascaded. Frightened, dread building and fingers pressed hard to my face, I couldn't take it anymore. Standing up, I crossed to the deck rail, and at the top of my lungs, head thrown back, I screamed and swore at the sea – again and again – until the fear was gone.

I found an entrance to the inside of the ship, and in the warmth and presence of others, my circumstances didn't seem quite so dire. But, even with a mind thinking more rationally, the absurdity of the trip was startling. In the space of approximately one month, I was supposed to find a place to live, apply to and be accepted at a medical school, and learn a foreign language (not just to gain conversational facility, but so I could understand lectures and read medical texts!).

Just go through the motions, I decided. *Get through these next few weeks, end the madness, and go home.*

FRANCE AND MONSIEUR L'ABBE

Around 2:00 a.m. I arrived in Dieppe, and after some delay, boarded the night train to Paris. All the coaches I had traveled on in Ireland, England, and now France, seemed to be redolent of similar odors: sweating bodies, cigarette smoke, oranges, grapes, and cheese. Seats were not available. I found a space on the floor just beyond the men's room at the end of the car. On the bright side, no one was walking over me; on the not-so-bright side, each time the lavatory door opened, the stench was overpowering.

We arrived at the Gare St. Lazare train station in Paris in the early morning. A vast enclosure, its glassed arch extended over a series of tracks lined with trains whose whistle shrieks rebounded off the walls as they arrived and departed. Crowds of people filled the platforms. As I made my way toward the central terminal, the hysterical fear of the previous evening on the ship became a reality. I was completely unable to communicate: an extraordinary feeling of being totally alone and helpless. Thank God I had a piece of paper with an address. What would I have done without it?

After pointing out my destination to various uniformed individuals, I eventually found the proper queue, and after exchanging pounds for francs, purchased my ticket to Val d'Or. The town was about thirty minutes southeast of Paris. After stops along the outskirts of the city, the commuter train arrived at the Val d'Or station about mid-morning. Quite easily, I found the Avenue de Longchamps and the house, a two-story stucco affair, situated half-way down a hill at the bottom of what I presumed to be the River Seine. The Eiffel Tower was visible a great distance away.

An older lady responded to my knock. "Bonjour, Monsieur," she said. Again I produced the address and pointed to the name.

66

"Oui; Monsieur L'Abbe habite ici mais il depart pour la matin." She pointed to a time on her watch. My understanding was that Father Wright lived there and was away for the morning.

The lady invited me into the house, brought me to a parlor, which was very cool, and pointed to a seat. I sat down and promptly fell asleep.

When I awoke, a man was sitting in front of me, smoking a cigarette. Bespectacled, middle-aged, with a balding pate, he wore black trousers and a short-sleeved black shirt with a white clerical collar. Introductions were made, during which I mentioned to Father the lady in Edinburgh who provided his name and address.

"Can't place her at all," he responded, "but I'm delighted she remembered me – and that you found your way here."

Concerning accommodations, he indicated the main house was full, but a sunroom in the front of the dwelling should be adequate. I told him I'd be happy with that, made arrangements for payment and settled in.

Later, I discussed with Father the reason for my trip and gave a summary of my progress, or the lack thereof. Citing my lack of enthusiasm for the project, I indicated the impetus derived from an aunt who had high expectations for me. A recent conversation with her, I said, convinced me to finish the course since the issue would be resolved, one way or the other, in the next few weeks. Listening intently, Father Wright surprised me with his reaction. Rather than agreeing with me and dismissing the whole plan as farfetched, he displayed enthusiasm for the endeavor. An Aunt Bertha in clerical clothing!!

"I'll do what I can to help," he said. "I do have some connections at the Sorbonne. But, to be very candid, the language issue is a major obstacle."

The following day I met my housemates. They included a Frenchman, probably in his mid-twenties, who worked for a TV station and spoke English well. Part of his job, he told me, was checking equipment at the top of the Eiffel Tower. He had a neat sports car, and as I would later learn, an equally neat girl friend. Also in the house was an American couple on vacation; a US Army Sergeant attached to a local American military facility, and two Frenchmen who worked in a button factory.

My first evening there, the factory workers took me out to supper – as a welcoming gesture – and although the conversation didn't exactly flow, we had a good time. I was most appreciative of their hospitality.

A Renaissance Man

Autocratic in bearing and formal in speech, Father Wright was an interesting chap. An Anglican minister who converted to Catholicism, he had been Pastor of the local parish for four years. Aside from his native English, he was fluent in French and Spanish. He celebrated daily Mass in a small stone chapel, a couple of blocks from the house. (On occasion I would come to assist him.) Attendance was sparse; the congregation consisted of seven or eight women, and every now and then, an elderly gentleman.

After Mass one morning, we walked around what Father described as an upper-middle-class neighborhood; most of the residents commuted to their jobs in Paris. Father explained that the absence of activity around the homes was a consequence of the summer exodus of families to the cooler south. The village of Val d'Or was a collection of small shops at the base of the hill, across from the Seine. Beyond rose the Bois de Boulogne, a two thousand acre park, formerly a hunting preserve for royalty, now a pastoral refuge for city-worn Parisians.

Over the next weeks, Father Wright and I traveled to Paris on a few occasions. Well versed in architecture, sculpture, painting, and literature, he was an excellent guide. We visited the usual tourist attractions: the Sacré-Coeur with the small chapel adjoining, Montmartre, Place Pigalle, and the Tuillieres among others. But he also took me to back streets and little known sections of the city, all with their own history. One afternoon was spent at the Louvre. Father possessed not only extraordinary knowledge of the technical aspects of the compositions, but the subtext of the paintings as well: the circumstances of the artist at the time of the work, who the people in the painting were, their relationships to the artist, and the significance of each setting. After our jaunts, we stopped for coffee and a croissant before heading home. This gave Father the opportunity to review the highlights of the day and question me as if I were a student. I enjoyed it thoroughly.

As he had mentioned, Father Wright had contacts at the Sorbonne. On the morning of August 22 we met with the Assistant Dean of the medical school. Father had translated my college documents into French. The Dean was helpful but not particularly optimistic. He felt it would take at least a year to learn French well enough to be successful in the medical program. Nevertheless I filled out an application. The tuition for one year was $63; classes began on November 3rd.

The priest was extremely helpful; nothing could have been accomplished without his assistance. However, I started to develop an uneasy feeling. Not a specific event, small things: inappropriate compliments, occasional touches, which though probably inadvertent, were disquieting.

THE PANTHÉON

Time was running out. Now late August, the outlook was bleak, with nothing, save the Sorbonne, considered hopeful. The inclination to write Aunt Bertha and rehash the old arguments was rejected: been there, done that.

Mainly to preserve the appearance of effort, I enrolled on August 29th in a language program at the Panthéon, a branch of the Sorbonne, geared specifically to foreign students in situations such as mine. Immersion in the language was advertised, to establish a level of fluency adequate to the demands of the Sorbonne curriculum. If it proved to be inadequate I could say, in good conscience, that I tried, and finally the last nail could be struck in the coffin of "the project."

Five mornings a week I took a bus from the village to the Metro at Pont de St. Cloud, then on to Paris. The bus was great fun: jammed with people - many hanging out the windows and off the back of the vehicle - on their way to work. Shouting back and forth, they enjoyed a repartee totally meaningless to me. Since generally the same people took the same bus each morning, I soon became a regular and it wasn't long before I heard, "Bonjour Yank," and attempts were made to draw me into conversation. I found the French to be extremely friendly.

A COUNTRY BLESSED

During that summer of 1955, no matter where I traveled, being American seemed to confer a certain cachet. Conversations with an assortment of people made me realize the perception most had of the United States: a vast land blessed with extraordinary abundance, the leader of the world economically and militarily, a country that set the bar in entertainment, movies, music, fashion, and quality of life. To a large extent that was true during the post WW II era. By virtue of my accidental birth in the United States, I was part of the picture they imagined, painted with the same brush. My opinion was sought on a variety of topics, and my answers, even if not always accepted, were listened to with interest and not dismissed out of hand. The attention given was sometimes obvious but even when nuanced, there was no mistaking it. Probably a stretch, but perhaps this is how the citizens of Rome were viewed when that empire was in its heyday.

Persevering (If Nothing Else)

Those mornings, on arrival in Paris, I breakfasted on croissants and Espresso at a small café in the shadow of the Pantheon dome. Often I bought the *Herald Tribune* (Paris edition, written in English), found a bench in the small park across the street, and caught up on the news.

Class met for two hours. Approximately 15 people enrolled, of mixed ethnicities: Greek, Spanish, British, German, and Saudi Arabian. Lunch was in a large student cafeteria, the French Alliance; the food was excellent and inexpensive. Afternoons, I walked about the city endeavoring to translate signs and advertisements and decipher the chatter of passersby. In a café or shop, as though contemplating a purchase, I attempted conversations. American movies with French subtitles were helpful.

Evenings in the house were spent studying until supper, which I often ate at a local café with the two workers from the button factory. A family atmosphere prevailed. Wives and children stayed in the restaurant section while the men played cards or darts in the bar. Everyone was pleasant to me, the only foreigner in the place. English was not spoken, and with my limited fluency, my evening meal was limited to beef steak and red wine for quite some time. My button factory friends got me a job with them two afternoons a week. No skill was required, and it exposed me to the language, while I earned a few francs.

For a short period I became very homesick. Even the Fisherman's Co-Op was remembered with nostalgia. Letters from Bertha or my father and mother became a lifeline. Maria's letters were eagerly anticipated. She felt joining me in Paris for a few days would make for a great reunion. For reasons that escape me now, it never happened. Her letters, however, which I still have, eased my celibate void. Eventually the lonely mood passed and I returned to my usual mildly depressed state.

A Classical Music Buff

Through my assisting at Mass with Father, I became friendly with a couple of families in the village of Val d'Or. One or the other of the families usually invited me to supper once a week. Each family had a teenage son and the three of us often went out for a couple of beers afterwards and shot some pool. They were both about three years younger than I and were in love with everything American. Neither could wait until he was old enough to visit the US.

One night we went to a festival on the bank of the Seine, near the Pont de St Cloud. While walking home, we were joined by an older man, who during the ensuing conversation, learned I was American. Small talk followed which included his introduction: Herbert Fox, retired architect.

"I hope," he said to me, "that you're being treated well; the Americans were very decent to me when I lived there."

"Everyone's been very helpful," I assured him.

Herbert went on to inform us that he had studied for a time in Chicago, admired Frank Lloyd Wright, and wished that the French architectural community could be as imaginative as their colleagues in the states. He seemed like a pleasant enough fellow, and when in the course of our parting remarks, he invited me to meet the following Sunday, "to show you my neighborhood in Paris," I assumed it another instance of payback for hospitality enjoyed in the U.S. I accepted the offer.

On the appointed day, since the weather was mild, we walked the length of the Champs Elysses, then attended the movie "Desiree," followed by supper at a very nice restaurant. Interesting guy, this Herbert Fox: retired, once married, since divorced, seemingly intelligent, and he fancied himself a classical music buff. Herbert didn't smoke or drink. At the end of the evening he suggested we meet again the following week at his apartment.

"I would love to introduce you to my Brahms and Beethoven collection."

Thinking about it later, second thoughts intruded, and I decided not to keep the appointment. Although probably well-intentioned, Herbert was too smooth and sophisticated for a country boy like me; Ludwig and Johannes would have to wait.

A NIGHT TO REMEMBER

The American couple staying at the house, Ben and Eva (real names forgotten), invited me to join them for a night on the town – their final "blow-out before heading back to the states." They both taught at a college in the mid-west and classes were beginning in a few weeks.

"I'm very complimented to be included in your last hurrah," I told them. "Sure."

After sampling a string of bistros, we made our way to the famous Lido, renowned for their topless dancers, and where Josephine Baker, the black American entertainer, beloved in Paris (and one of the singers on "Cabaret Night in Paris"), used to perform. After we agreed that it was too pricey, too commercial, and too full of tourists, we decided to move on to less exotic fare. A club within walking distance, a few blocks from the bustle of the Champs Elysse, that might be more our style was suggested.

Located in the basement of an unimposing building, on a narrow side street, the place offered no pretense of glamour - but we found music that made our night. A series of open windows ran below the ceiling, just above sidewalk level. On the opposite wall was a haphazard arrangement of faded black and white photographs of musicians and bands. It was something of a crash pad for entertainers after their shows: a place to have a few drinks, smoke a little pot (very available in those days), and jam with whomever might be around.

Ten or twelve tables were scattered about the room, couches along the wall, with a bar at the back. Including our group there were about fifteen people in attendance. At the head of the room was a quartet - piano, trumpet, saxophone and banjo - playing Dixieland. Eschewing the brassy and percussive, their offerings were laid back: a down-and-dirty blues style. There weren't any set pieces, the melodies just flowed one to the other. The four meshed seamlessly, obviously having a good time doing what they did best. We learned later that they played with the Sidney Bechet orchestra, a group out of New Orleans, who were very big in France at the time. Sidney, who played soprano sax, and Josephine Baker, the chanteuse, both arrived in Paris in the mid-twenties where each found their niche and a popularity neither had realized in the States.

Eva leaned toward me. "Do you like this kind of music?" she asked.

"Love it," I answered. I explained my taste was acquired back in Holy Cross when a college mate occasionally corralled a few of us to head to New York (where he lived) to hit the clubs. "That's where the seed was sown. Eventually I became partial to bands that came out of Chicago and New Orleans during the 1920s and early 30s. You know, guys like Bix Beiderbecke, Jack Teagarden, Jelly Roll Morton - wonderful stuff."

"So you won't be bored if we hang out here for awhile?"

I laughed. "I think we've found a home."

Ben and Eva were into the moment. Both were musically inclined and had actually met while rehearsing a show - he played piano in the college band and Eva sang. They sat holding hands as if mesmerized. At times, one leaned toward the other and whispered; the other nodded in response. As I watched, I couldn't help but be struck by how well they seemed to fit. They complimented each other in so many areas: intelligence, humor, travel compatibility, looks, and now music. I couldn't imagine getting that lucky.

As night moved towards dawn, the room, turgid with smoke and the acrid hint of cannabis, became crowded; musicians relinquished their seats to others. Well into our third bottle of wine, we closed the place around 3:00 a.m.

"The best night of music I think I've ever had in my life," was how Ben summed up the experience.

"For once, big guy," Eva responded, "I agree with you."

Grey fissures streaked the sky to the east as we made our way back into the city. We strolled along the Seine, revisiting the events of the night, in no hurry to go home. A passerby pointed out an all-night café where, with Notre Dame framed in the window, we had coffee and croissants.

As we crossed the Pont Neuf on the way to the Metro (the Parisian subway), Ben suddenly stopped.

"Goddammit," he announced. "We've got to do something symbolic, something memorable to remember our last night, this incredible last night."

"Well, honey…," said Eva, pointing to the river, its inky surface dappled streetlight-orange, "you could always jump in the Seine. That would be memorable."

"Very funny," he replied.

"But," she continued, "if you're not going to do that, maybe we could each throw in a coin and make a wish – one for all of us."

We agreed that was a great idea.

"But what will it be?" I asked.

"How about that we all meet in Paris again someday?" Eva suggested.

"Yes!" said Ben. "That's it. And we'll all stay in touch."

"Let's do it," said Eva. So with great ceremony, we raised our coins. "Revoir, Paris!" shouted out Eva.

"Revoir, Paris," we shouted back.

And with that we threw the shiny pieces high into the air and watched until their glitter was lost in the darkness below. Then arm-in-arm we strode off the bridge into the fading night, laughing uproariously as we attempted to sing the first bars of the "Marseilles."

So ended our night to remember.

(We never stayed in touch; the wish made in our wine-sodden state was never realized. However, on flights to Paris over the years, I've always found my way to the Pont Neuf to drop a coin into the Seine, in remembrance of that evening with Ben and Eva. On occasion I've used another mode of transport – less expensive and requiring no passport. Settled onto a sofa, with a goblet of wine at the ready, I haul out a Sidney Bechet CD, and before eight bars of "Si Tu Vois Ma Mere" have been played, I'm returned to the sights, smells, and sounds of a Paris night in 1955.)

Although I was dismissive of my progress with French, the locals assured me I was doing well. To increase my exposure, Father assigned me the grocery shopping for the house. Each evening we conversed in French for one half hour, and each day I translated a section of the newspaper. Little by little, I started to better understand TV ads and greater portions of conversation. I was still far removed from the facility required for medical school.

I became uncomfortable in the house. My discomfort related to an incident which occurred in late August, a particularly warm, late summer night. Father Wright had the room next to mine, and during the night I heard the connecting door open.

"Gene," Father asked, "Are you managing all right?"

I started to get up but Father quickly came over and sat on the edge of the bed.

"Sorry to bother," he continued, "but was worried about you; damned heat's oppressive. I've an extra fan if you want it."

"No, I'm all set, Father. Thanks anyway." The room was in semi-darkness, with only street lights providing illumination, but it appeared Father was wearing a gown of some sort.

While he sat on the edge of the bed, we engaged in small talk: mosquitoes, humidity and the cooler weather which would be arriving soon. The Father started to rub my shoulders while he commented on how much "joy" I had brought to the house, how he admired my efforts to learn French, and what a "nice" boy I was. Acutely uncomfortable, I didn't move and said nothing. Then his soft, sweaty hand was on the small of my back and fingers were being inserted beneath the waist band of my shorts. I pushed his hand away and stood up.

"Father, I'm tired; need to get some sleep."

"I know you do, Gene. I was just concerned and thought we

could chat awhile."

With my background, what was happening blew my mind. But what really got me was the change in his voice. The Father's usually stern, crisply authoritative tone was soft, whiney, almost pleading as he insisted that he just wanted to talk. We could talk, I told him, in the morning. Father left the room.

The incident was never mentioned to Aunt Bertha or my father. They would never fault a priest and probably would have told me that I was misinterpreting a friendly gesture, that I should be more appreciative of his concern. Indeed, I was very appreciative of the Father and had no problem with his sexual preferences as long as they didn't include me. However, I knew at that point my days at Avenue De Longchamps were numbered. Father was leaving with some friends on a hiking trip to England and Wales the following week. He asked if I wished to come along. I declined.

At Father's request, I continued to assist him at morning mass before heading to Paris. Although we were both aware of the awkward situation, it wasn't apparent to anyone else. Father's demeanor was unchanged, and if it weren't for my vivid recollection of his damp touch and maudlin behavior of a few nights earlier, one might think it all a bad dream. After Mass the morning of his departure, as we walked together back to the house, he very quietly asked, "I hope we can still be friends?" He looked at me closely. I nodded "yes" in response.

My feeling then (as now): the sexual proclivities of a priest, whether of a homosexual or heterosexual bent, were of little concern. One goes to Mass for the song, not the singer, and once you make the messenger a part of the equation that defines your faith, you have taken the first step to losing it.

My attitude about my mission, however, changed somewhat around this time. The whole medical school project had begun as a lark, a fun thing to do for the summer. And although nothing had occurred to pique my interest, a considerable effort, nevertheless, had been made to effect a successful outcome. Bertha certainly provided the impetus and enthusiasm; I had done the legwork and suffered the rejections; and more recently, Father Wright had lent his support. Realizing these efforts, the distance traveled, and the money spent, to come up empty-handed would be, despite my antipathy to the undertaking, a disappointment.

After French class one day, I stopped by the American Express office in Paris. Aunt Bertha preferred that address for her correspondence; she felt it more reliable. In fact, there was a letter from her. The front page was basically a weather report:

...a marvelous Indian summer. The water is still warm and delightful for swimming. A recent storm cleared the air of humidity and the trees of most of their leaves - looks like an early winter.

There was a paragraph or two more, and then a surprising P.S. after her usual closing:

Love and God Bless,
P.S. Look on the back—

When I turned the sheet over, I found the following:

You have been accepted at the Royal College of Surgeons in Ireland, with classes to begin October 1st.
Congratulations,
Bert and Dad

I was stunned. Needing to sit down, I found a chair on the opposite side of the room. There I sat, elbows on knees, rereading those few lines again and again. It was mid-September, the twelfth hour, hope all but gone - now, this incredible news. The whole thing was beyond belief.

The immediate physical sensation was one of relief; in those few minutes, weight carried for weeks lifted from my shoulders. And winning the battle, beating the odds - alarms sounding notwithstanding - was an awesome feeling. But since I was basically only along for the ride, the day really belonged to my aunt. For me, the real joy of the moment was the pleasure and vindication this acceptance would give her. I raised my head toward the ceiling, and said in a fairly loud voice, "Thank you, God." With that, a man sitting across from me, eyed me rather strangely, stood up and walked away. A little bit later I headed off.

Lightheaded and euphoric I wandered the streets, eventually finding a bench overlooking the Seine. The breeze off the gray river was cool. Hints of fall were about: the light more sharp, the stroll of tourists less languid, book kiosks were boarded; spirals of brown leaves pirouetted down the empty sidewalk. A quick puff of breeze induced a shiver of apprehension. With shirt collar turned up and hands shoved deep in my pockets, the cold reality of what this acceptance implied began to take hold.

Starting October 1st, I would be entering a program in which I had no interest. According to the Surgeon's brochure, I also might be required to repeat science courses before being accepted into the medical school proper. For four years at Holy Cross they had been the bane of my existence – go through them again? That was not a fate I wished to endure a second time. It was an impossible situation. Although I had never indicated to Bertha or my father a desire to become a physician, I let the process begin. A momentum had developed which I felt sure would falter given the time constraint. It hadn't. Now, with an acceptance in hand, I couldn't suddenly opt out. At that point there was no way to extract myself from this self-inflicted predicament. The only option: go with the flow.

O ver the next two days I prepared to leave. The tenant, who worked at the local US Army facility, typed up and sent a very official-looking letter to the USAF requesting a deferment from my active duty assignment, for the purpose of attending medical school (which was approved). One of the families in town had a small party for me. The people I worked with in the button factory gave me a bottle of wine which we opened and drank on the spot. Father Wright, back from his trip, had a get-together at the house. Somewhat awkwardly, but sincerely, I thanked him for all he had done. At the end of the evening Father took me aside. Knowing of my disinterest in medicine, he told me, "Be patient, for God works in strange ways. He certainly has in my life and maybe he will in yours." I asked the Father to include me in his prayers. He said he would.

Au revoir Val d'Or. For the last time, I took the bus to the Metro and on to Gare St. Lazare, remembering my arrival a few weeks ago. I enjoyed a comfortable train ride to Dieppe where I boarded the ferry to Dover. I had written Maria that I would visit her in Edinburgh before going on to Dublin.

An incident on the boat to England illustrated how my background still influenced me. While in conversation with a very attractive girl on deck, an announcement was made that a Catholic Mass was being celebrated someplace on the ship. The girl indicated, in so many words, her disdain for Catholics. She hoped I was not one of "them." If she hadn't been so good looking, I probably would have admitted my affiliation. But she was. "Of course not," was my reply. Immediately I thought of Peter denying Jesus, but I figured if Peter had two more shots at redemption, I did also.

Maria was excited to see me. After reminiscences over drinks and dinner we went back to her place. It was as if I had never left. In the morning we took the tram to the train station and made plans to keep in touch. Her modeling contract finished in a couple of weeks, and she said that she would love to visit Dublin before heading back to Paris. Somehow I think we both knew this was not likely to happen - and it didn't. Instead, a kiss, a long embrace on the platform, a final wave as the train pulled away. Coincidentally, the husband and wife who managed the small bar Maria and I frequented were also on the train, going to Blackpool for a holiday.

(Many years later, in 2009, I returned to Edinburgh and found the bed and breakfast where Maria and I had met. The interior of the house was being refurbished but a worker let me walk around. Incredibly, that particular day, the wall between our two rooms in the basement was being torn down. As I poked about in the plaster and debris, I was almost certain I heard a woman's voice, scarcely a whisper. "J'attendrai," it said. "Le jour et la nuit, J'attendrai toujours…" Photos were taken…a nostalgic moment.)

On the train that morning, I marveled at how my life had changed. Just two months earlier, I was cutting fish at the Point Judith Fisherman's Co-Op; now I was headed to medical school in Ireland. So much had happened in the interim: Ireland with its beauty and friendliness, the melancholy of Liverpool, the vitality of Edinburgh, Maria, the French experience, and Monsieur L'Abbe. And now, the next chapter… Apprehensive, I felt uncertain where this path would lead. But, on this day at least, the sun was out and all seemed right with the world. I decided to leave whatever was to happen in the lap of the Gods.

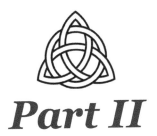

Part II

L iverpool, bleak and sunless, unchanged from my previous recollection, was scarcely noticed as I was soon aboard a B&I steamer. Easing past the Royal Liver Building, through the interminable locks, we made our way to the open sea. Although the high tourist season had ended weeks earlier, the ship was full: all available benches and seats occupied. Bunked on an inside deck, a surprisingly placid Irish Sea allowed fitful sleep until landfall in Dublin.

Cold wind and a gray sun glinting off a sullen Liffey River welcomed our early morning arrival. Tired, dirty and hungry, I began the trek to the city center along sidewalks teeming with men headed to work on the docks. Walking against the tide of bodies, I was forced to take refuge inside a recessed store entrance - Kilmartin Turf Accountant - until the crowds thinned.

When I eventually reached O'Connell Street, the wide expanse bisecting the city, I stopped to get my bearings. Apparently my indecision was noted; a voice suddenly interrupted.

"Hey Mister, need some help?" A gnarled little fellow with a tanned, wrinkled face and a stack of newspapers under his arm, approached.

"I guess I do. I'm starting school at the College of Surgeons and need to find someplace to live around there."

"Och," he said, "Surgeons. Then you'll be needing the number 9 bus. Hop off at Lesson Street near Stephens Green. Plenty of places around there."

"Thanks for your help." I gave him the change I had in my pocket.

"So you're going to be a doctor are you?" he continued. "Oh, that's a fine place you're going. Lots of foreigners there, you know... blacks. But I like them. Not snobby like Trinity." The man had a heavy accent and with lips tight around a cigarette, was difficult to understand. "Anyway, good luck to you. Hope you enjoy Dublin and...oh, here's your bus coming. So... off ya go."

(Over the next two years, I occasionally ran into him at his usual spot near the O'Connell Bridge. Curious as to my progress, he seemed genuinely pleased when I told him "pretty well." Our short chats always included his admonitions to study hard, not drink too much, and to "be careful of the girls." His concern felt almost fatherly, as if discovering this lost soul straight off the boat, he wanted to be sure he remained on course. One day, as I traveled over the bridge on a bus, my friend wasn't in his usual spot. I never saw him again. I never knew his name.)

Traffic, more bicycles than cars, jammed the intersection at Lesson Street and St. Stephens Green. The morning was crisp and cool, the air sharpened by the smell of peat. A restaurant was found where my empty belly was filled, and with energy restored, the search was begun for a place to stay. Without much difficulty I found a room, for one night only, at the nearby Pembroke House. Although more expensive than expected, it allowed me a place to deposit my bag and clean up before seeking more reasonable accommodations.

My first stop, however, was the College of Surgeons, on the opposite side of the Green. A preregistration year was required before one could enter the medical school proper. This I wanted to avoid, as not only would I have to take science courses again, which weren't my strong suit, but more importantly, another year would be added to an already five-year program.

I made an appointment to see the registrar, a Mr. Rae, for the following day. I hoped I'd be persuasive enough at the meeting to negotiate an exemption. When I asked the lady who gave me the appointment to describe his temperament, she allowed he could be "crusty" at times, but always fair in his dealings with students. She also informed me that the young lady who had been so helpful on my earlier visit had left for a job in the city.

With that business accomplished, I sought a permanent place to stay. Premises that took in tenants were not advertised in most cases, so I selected houses at random. If a room was not available, leads for other places were often given by the landlords. With two colleges in the area and classes set to start within the week, it became apparent that I'd be lucky to find anything in the Surgeons neighborhood. The last landlady, who offered her sympathy but little else, suggested Hyde House, located nearby on Adelaide Road. She pointed out a narrow street, Hatch Lane, at the end of which I would find the place.

"Hyde House" was stenciled into a stained glass fanlight above the door. A red-brick Victorian facade was fronted by tall, curtained windows which reflected trees along the street. The door bell, a large key centered in a wide wooden door, sounded deep inside the house.

A short, stout woman, wearing an apron and smoking a cigarette, opened the door. "Yes, Mister? What can I do for you?"

I told her that I was starting school in Dublin and needed a place to stay. "A lady the next street over said that you might have room," I explained.

"Nothing here," came her quick reply. "And not much you'll find around here. Not this time of year." The words came in short bursts, her lips hardly moving. Then she began to close the door.

"Maybe," I said quickly, "something temporary, while I look around?"

She hesitated. "There's a small parlor. Only has a couch."

"That'll do fine," I replied. "How much do you charge?"

She threw away her cigarette. "Three pounds ten a week, full board, two pounds seven, partial," she replied.

"What's partial?" I asked.

"No noon meals except Sunday."

I made a quick calculation. That was less than ten dollars a week. "Partial's fine," I said.

Still standing on the steps outside the door, the landlady's hand was raised, shielding her eyes from the sun. Aware of the annoyance, I asked if she wanted to step inside. I followed her into a dim foyer where a brocade rug, hanging along one wall, was reflected in a large mirror on the opposite side.

"First," she stated, "there are rules."

I nodded.

"Rent's due in advance. No credit," she added. "No female guests at any time. No guests, male or female, after tea. Breakfast's at seven, tea at six. Nothing held beyond fifteen minutes. No drinking in the rooms. You drink?"

"A little," I replied.

"Then drink outside. A hot bath...three days notice." She paused before wrapping up with, "That's about all for now."

I continued to nod my assent during this exchange but began to question my choice. I felt sure that any number of monasteries would be more flexible.

"That's fine," I told her. "I'll bring my things by in the morning and pay for the week."

"Do you want to see where you'll be staying?" she asked.

I shook my head "no" and indicated that I was sure it would be fine. She extended her hand. "My name is Miss Halligan." I noticed a trace of a smile.

"Nice to meet you, Miss Halligan," I replied, and shook her hand. "I'm Gene McKee."

"Welcome to Hyde House, Mr. McKee."

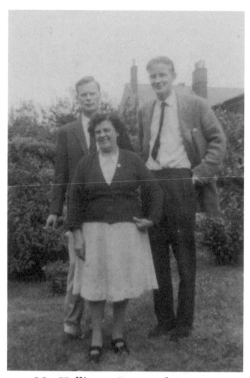

Ms. Halligan, Gene and Eugene
O'Connell, Med Student from Cork

Little did I know, on that September morning in 1955, that I would be associated with this little woman for my entire career in Dublin.

The College of Surgeons was a large, gray, stolid structure facing St. Stephen's Green. One of the People's Army strategic locations during the 1916 Easter uprising against the British, the exterior of the building was pock-marked, as a result of receiving rounds of shot during the fighting. My appointment with Professor Rae, the registrar, was conducted in the room from which, reputedly, the Countess Markiewicz, a loyalist who married a Polish count, commanded the rebel operations for that section of Dublin.

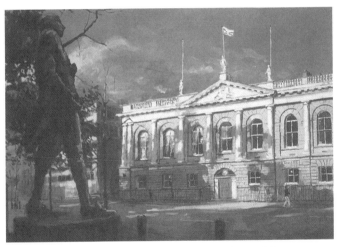

The Royal College of Surgeons in Dublin

A gray-haired, avuncular appearing gentleman, glasses perched on the tip of his nose, Professor Rae listened attentively to my petition. He had something of a bemused expression on his face, as one would who had heard the song before but yet remained open to any novel variations. When I finished he indicated his appreciation of the fact that I had passed the subjects required in the pre-registration year. Unfortunately he was adamant that an exception could not be made that would allow me to skip the year and directly enter the medical school proper.

"First, it would set a precedent which I do not want to have to deal with in the future," Professor Rae said. "And...you are American. We would not want to give the impression that you were able to buy your way out of the requirement."

The latter brought a smile to my face.

"I will tell you, however, that I believe you would be our first student from the United States; something of a distinction, I would think, and a milestone for the College. But that's neither here nor there. Mr. McKee, you need to make a decision. Classes are set to start within the week. Either you enroll now and accept the pre-registration year, or your place will be given to someone else. So, what's it to be?"

"Give me a moment, Sir?" I asked. My mind raced. The choice could not be more stark. Go home and suffer my aunt's displeasure or waste another year slogging through the detested sciences. Bertha will eventually get over it, I reasoned. Plus, I'll be in Texas in three weeks, faraway from R.I. So let's get this hair-brained scheme done with now. The Professor glanced at his watch and arranged some papers on his desk.

After another moment Mr. Rae folded his hands and looked directly at me. "Well?"

"Sir," I began, "I think..." and then paused.

"Think what?" he asked.

I took a deep breath. "That I would like to join the class."

"Well done, Mr. McKee. Welcome to the College of Surgeons."

We shook hands.

Our first meeting was held in a large amphitheater - our primary classroom throughout the year. The class was comprised of 100 students, a fair number of whom were women. Most were from England and Ireland but I was surprised to see a large number of students of color. Subsequently, I learned they were from various parts of the Middle East, Far East and Africa. The College had established strong contacts with a number of countries in those areas and offered qualified candidates the chance of a medical education which they otherwise might not have had. As a result, Surgeons became, and has remained, a sought after medical school destination for students from those populations.

The College offered little in the way of social amenities. For the males, a common room was available which contained a snooker table, a leather couch, and a scattering of tables and chairs. Separate rooms were available for the ladies, where according to the College handbook: "careful provision is made for their comfort." Interplay between the sexes, aside from classroom activities, occurred either in the dining area - a large unadorned space containing a series of long tables and a well-worn upright piano (played with surprising facility by classmate Johnny Atkinson), or a stone-enclosed catacomb deep in the bowel of the building. Coffee, tea, sandwich rolls, and co-mingling were available there. In earlier times, the "Canteen," it was said, served as a holding area for cadavers prior to their final resting place in the anatomy theater.

Social divisions evolved in the class, largely determined by ethnicity. In the college setting, however, I was not aware of any overt discrimination. The same acceptance may not have been found in the general population of Dublin at the time. At Surgeons, those with similar cultures and origins seemed to naturally gravitate toward each other, staying within their group and comfort zone. Aside from sports teams, there were few social organizations which might encourage more college-wide participation. For those in my social circle, the pub was our forum and seldom would you see a person of color in the places we frequented. However, if they had chosen to join us, they would have undoubtedly been made most welcome.

A s the year progressed, I made friends. Among them was Pat O'Brien, who resided in digs nearby. Pat was from Gateshead, located in the northeast part of England, near Newcastle on Tyne. His father, a physician, had trained in Cork. A casual, relaxed demeanor effectively disguised Pat's keen intelligence and an unsuspected studiousness. At about 6 feet 4 inches, Pat towered over most of Dublin's population. On certain occasions, his stature grew when he demonstrated an ability to down a pint in something less than ten seconds - a handy feat should an un-believer wish to place a wager.

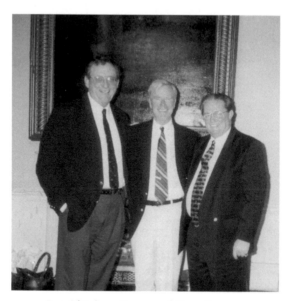

Pat O'Brien, Gene and Tom Lomas
at the Alumni Reunion of 2001 in Dublin

Another good friend was Tom Lomas. Tom looked as I thought a Britisher should: a sturdy, square build with erect carriage; confident demeanor; a mass of thick, black hair, neatly maintained; a somewhat defiant jaw; with sun-deprived English skin. Tom hailed from Macclesfield. More organized, studious and focused than either Pat or me, he did well scholastically, and at one point, was our class president and captain of our rowing team. Behind all the seriousness, however, lay a great sense of humor, and when primed with a pint or two of Guiness, he became as rowdy and raucous as the rest of the group.

Much of my time in Dublin revolved around my companionship with these two. We played rugby, crewed, crashed parties, acted in skits, drank copious quantities of stout, and at various times lived together. We also managed to pass a few exams along the way.

Life in the Digs

Hyde House was once the residence of Dr. Douglas Hyde, a poet and playwright, who founded the Gaelic League in the late 1800s. This organization sought to resurrect an Irish heritage slowly being extinguished by the English via their legislative majority and military dominance, with assistance from a complicit Catholic hierarchy. As a result of the league's efforts, the study of Gaelic was made part of the school curriculum, and traditional Irish sports (hurling and Gaelic football), were organized under the Gaelic Athletic Association. In literature and the theater, there was a similar resurgence of works done in the native tongue.

The digs worked out well. Within two weeks I had moved from my parlor to a proper room on the second floor, which included a roommate. Con Collins was from the west coast of Ireland and in his second year at University College Dublin, majoring in agriculture. After we became friendly, he confided to me his complete lack of interest in the field. At home, he lived with his parents and two younger brothers on a large farm. Being the oldest, he was expected to take over the management of the farm, upon either the demise of his father or his father's inability to manage it. The responsibility that would one day be his was a constant concern, but he soldiered on, mainly to not disappoint his father. (He left the digs within a few months. When I met him some time later, he was still pursuing his agricultural degree but also had achieved some resolution with his father and seemed more comfortable with his lot.)

Con and I shared a large room with two single beds. Two other rooms similar to ours and three single rooms made up the rental portion of the house. Miss Halligan's quarters were in the basement. The rooms had high ceilings with proportionately tall windows, which in the winter allowed large drafts of cold air inside - and the house lacked central heating. Each room was furnished with a set of drawers, a closet, and a cold water sink.

A large bathroom on the first floor contained the communal tub and a gas-fired water tank. It took three days to heat the bathwater, so a reservation system was in place. Only four or five of the tenants had to vie for spots, as half of the residents either had friends with baths, were involved with sports teams, or utilized public facilities in town. But for those of us still in the hunt, resourcefulness and luck were key. The situation often prompted a rather tense exchange with the landlady.

"Miss Halligan, I've got to take a bath."

"Lorna (one of the boarders) has it taken," would be the terse reply. "But if you like, I can put you down for the next opening."

"But that could be weeks away, Miss Halligan. I really need something before then."

She nodded. "I understand. The only thing I can suggest is talk to Lorna (or whoever was up next), and arrange something with her. Sometimes she visits friends and takes her bath there."

So that night at tea, I take Lorna (in this instance) aside and hopefully acquire her booking.

However, when finally in the tub for the big event, one discovered that the hot water didn't extend much above mid-thigh. Her frugality even extended to toilet paper. Local newspapers were cut into hand-size squares and attached to the commode wall. News of the recent past was read as snippets of unfinished sentences and broken paragraphs.

Partial board, as outlined by Miss Halligan, included breakfast and tea each day, with three meals on Sunday. The menu was quite regimented. Breakfast consisted of an egg, rasher, and blood pudding, preceded by a bowl of cereal: cold in the summer, warm in the winter. Wonderful homemade soda bread was available and rapidly consumed. Tea, served in small dented pots, was delicious. The evening repast consisted of meat, invariably lamb, with a vegetable, often Brussels sprouts – boiled until devoid of color and taste - and potatoes. Sunday's noon meal was similar but distinguished by a dessert, usually a trifle.

The digs were analogous to a boarding house in the States. Miss Halligan's possessed its own uniqueness, but it was typical of those existing in Dublin at the time. As with everything else, if you paid more, you could enjoy more of the creature comforts. Hyde House, I thought, was somewhere in the middle of the comfort spectrum. The clientele of the digs usually reflected its location. Those near the city were more likely to cater to working folk, whereas those near a college were populated mainly by students. At Hyde House, the split was fairly equal between students and working people. When I arrived, the tenants included three students; a retired, male principal; a postman; two shop girls; an older, single lady; and Miss Halligan's nephew.

An interesting dynamic became apparent as I settled into my new home. Although I have touted the friendliness I experienced in Ireland- in large part because of my nationality - I realized that in each instance the interactions were of a short duration - a meeting on a bus, a conversation on a roof, sitting at a bar - with the end of the relationship clearly in sight. At Hyde House, I was the only foreigner and I was going to be there long-term. There was a subtle resistance, especially on the part of the men, to become friendly. The implication: I was an intruder on their turf. I could tell that Con Collins wasn't happy to have me as a roommate initially, and it took him a long time to be comfortable with me. Maybe they thought I was depriving an Irishman of a place in a medical school, taking something that wasn't mine. Maybe it went back to the days "when the strangers came and tried to teach us their way." Also, it could have been my paranoia which I came by rightly. But I did find, for certain, that after I served my unspoken probation, during which their bias was allayed, a more amicable brand of Irishmen emerged.

THE PRINCIPAL

My initial impression of Frank Gillan, the retired school teacher and principal: a pompous, opinionated, boorish clod, and a dirty old man to boot. With the passage of weeks, then months, it dawned that his bluster and bravado were but a cover for the circumstances in which he now found himself. Once a somebody, a man of authority, the principal who demanded and received respect, he was slowly being entwined into the fabric of anonymity. As a drowning man would wave and shout for recognition, so did Frank. Chastened by the insight, I became less quick to judge the man behind the bombast.

In his late 60's, Frank was from Roscommon, scarcely visited since his move to Dublin some twenty-five years earlier. He had resided with Miss Halligan for over five years. Never married, his immediate family was deceased; his only relatives were a niece and nephew living in America. He was a heavy-set, big-boned man; his worn, craggy face, anchored by a prominent jaw, extended to a broad, bald dome. Gruff in speech and manner, with large hands more suited to manual labor, his appearance was at odds with the image usually associated with those in his profession.

Frank always seemed ready for class: clean-shaven with shirt and tie, sharpened pencil in his breast pocket, black shoes cut above the ankle and always shined. Reading the dictionary was his hobby; crossword puzzles, his relaxation; the constant cigarette, a sliver of white in a massive hand, his comfort.

Conversations with Frank turned on three basic themes: politics, education, and women. Politically, his views were unyielding. Fiercely, he opposed Fianna Fail, the party in power at the time, and their leader, Eamon DeValera – "a bloody blaggard who'll run this country into the ground." Frank's knowledge of government and Irish history was impressive, his interpretations imaginative. Historical conspiracies abounded at every turn with Frank. In his mind, for example, there was little doubt DeValera had orchestrated the ambush and death of Michael Collins, who had negotiated for peace with the British, at the cost of partition. His opinion, in this instance, was widely shared.

The educational system in Ireland was, according to Frank, in "a desperate state." Its decline and imminent demise being hastened, he'd insist, by influences as disparate as television, popular music, and corrupt government officials. Staunchly supportive of Gaelic being taught in the secondary school curriculum, he said one of the reasons he chose Hyde House as a residence was because of its association with Douglas Hyde.

Frank was also unyielding in his appraisals of the fairer sex. A committed bachelor, either by choice or good fortune, he expressed great hostility toward the institution of marriage: not the sacrament, but the stratagems employed by scheming women who lured men into their connubial web.

Without an audience available during the day, Frank's moment to expound on any of these subjects came when the tenants gathered before tea in the sitting room. During the winter months, Miss Halligan lit a fire using a mixture of peat and coke, around which the men of the house gathered, enjoying their cigarettes, while they discussed the news of the day. The women occupied a large couch and chairs placed against the opposite wall. As a cost-saving measure the fire was not maintained after tea.

If ladies were present, Frank confined his remarks to politics and educational matters. But if an all-male assembly - with little pretext, as if continuing a conversation already begun in his head - he would start. "Grind you down, they will. And bleed you dry while they're doing it."

"Who's that?" one would ask.

"Damn women." And he'd refer to a news item or something heard on the radio.

The small audience around the fire smiled and nodded. They had heard Frank's screed before.

"With their perfumes and tight skirts and God knows what else...," he'd continue, in his deep voice coarsened by cigarettes.

Dan Savage, another boarder, was adept at needling Frank, especially on the subject of women. With a wink to the rest of us, he'd begin.

"Why, you old bollocks, you'd give up your pension for a little bit of arse. My God, Frank, that's all you ever think about."

Grins stretched to laughs. Frank's face started to flush. Dan, like a picador circling his prey, poked and pierced with quick jabs of ridicule until Frank shook with agitation, his fleshy lips trembling.

"I could tell the lot of you a story or two," he'd say, his cigarette jerking up and down. "I know about women, had my share you know, back in Roscommon; plenty were after me."

"Oh, bullshit, Frank. You wouldn't know what to do if it were lying there twitching in front of you, you old fart."

And on it would go: Frank, deep crimson, almost blubbering, as he tried to convince us of his experience and virility. Dan hardly let him finish a sentence. The thrust, the parry, the palaver was all great fun.

Finally, time for tea and Dan would put his arm around Frank's shoulder. "Listen, you old bollocks, even though you ain't no Clark Gable, we like you anyway." Soon that craggy face found a smile and all was well.

However, if a young female boarder were to strike up a conversation with Frank, his face would light up, a grin stretched from ear to ear. "Why, aren't you looking grand this evening, Miss?" he'd say, offering a cigarette. "From Bandon are you? And a beautiful place it is. Visited there years ago. Tell me, do the Flynns still have a pub there?" And on he would go, delighted with her company. Of course, when the young lady left, he would lean over to whoever was there and begin, in his hoarse whisper, "Right tart that one. Did you see her looking me over? Sure, I know her people. Chancers, the whole lot of them." Finding his stride he'd proceed to skewer the family and forecast the dire outcome for the unfortunate man who became involved with "that one."

Frank enjoyed the digs and its small community. Taking an interest in all of us, he took time to listen to our frustrations with school or work. Curious, he asked about backgrounds and families; sympathetic, he consoled when exams were failed, opportunities missed or jobs lost. We were his only social contact, as visitors, letters, and phone calls were absent. Even his tutoring opportunities had passed. An enduring image remains: passing by the sitting room in mid-day, Frank alone, seated in a hard-backed chair, all dressed up, reading his dictionary, as though waiting for his class to return from lunch - and there he would stay all day.

UCD (University College Dublin)

A particular advantage of Hyde House was its location, approximately two blocks from UCD and its medical library. Since Pat O'Brien and Tom Lomas also lived nearby, we often met there around 7:00 p.m. In the winter, it was too cold to study in the digs, while the library offered a more comfortable atmosphere. Since we were not students at UCD, we had no right to use their facility, but we were never challenged; it became a haunt for years.

Our exit strategy on those nights was to depart the library, just before 10 o'clock, and sprint to McGrath's pub at the corner of Leeson Street, about a block away. At that time in Ireland, pubs closed in the winter at 10 o'clock. But if one gained admittance before that time, you were good for at least fifteen to twenty minutes. Joe, the proprietor, started calling "time" some fifteen minutes before closing, but his attempts to clear the place before 10:30 p.m. seldom proved successful. So after a chat and a pint of stout, we headed back to the digs and to bed.

Through these excursions to the library and contacts made through the digs, I met many UCD students over the years, from all parts of Ireland. They included the wealthy, the not so wealthy, and farmer's sons and daughters; the common denominator was their ability to qualify for entrance to the college. (Tuition was insignificant as it was a government-funded institution. Their charter was to train students in areas beneficial both to the student and to Ireland's economic growth. The main courses offered included engineering, law, agriculture, and medicine.)

The Newman Chapel was another UCD facility which Tom, Pat and I utilized. Located across from St. Stephens Green, it derived its name from Cardinal Henry Newman, a convert to Catholicism, one of the original rectors at UCD and considered one of the Catholic Church's greatest theologians. A pleasant, little chapel with seating capacity for perhaps a hundred parishioners, it was our church of choice most Sundays. We sat in the balcony, usually suffering from varying degrees of distress and distemper, secondary to the previous night's activities. A highlight of the service was the superb voice of a tenor who regularly sang there. To this day, excepting the great Beniamino Gigli, I have never heard a better rendition of "Panis Angelicus."

After the service, we moved on to a local coffee shop, deconstructed the previous night's activities and shared the *Manchester Guardian* newspaper. Although none of us aspired to a moral life (the converse more apt), we all managed to make Mass on most Sundays - a tenuous connection maintained more from habit than holiness.

One afternoon on Grafton Street, amongst the crowd, I recognized Tom Conneen, a fellow graduate from my 1955 Holy Cross class. Although in the same program, we never had any social interaction. Tom informed me that he had started his first year of medical school at Trinity. After a pleasant conversation we agreed to meet sometime for a drink. Although somewhat chagrined to hear that he hadn't been required to complete a preregistration year, I learned later that he had been working on his application for over a year, whereas mine had evolved over a matter of weeks.

Trinity was, and remains, the oldest and most prestigious college in Dublin. The course structure, similar to that found in traditional English universities such as Cambridge and Oxford, offered Bachelor of Arts degrees in either the humanities or science. Many graduates achieved fame and occasional infamy, most prominently: Samuel Becket and Oscar Wilde. The American, J.P. Donleavy, achieved considerable acclaim for *The Ginger Man*, a fictionalized account of a student's time in Dublin during the late 1940s. Donleavy studied at Trinity on the American GI bill, but left before obtaining a degree.

The student population was predominately English with a secondary contingent from the continent. Tom Conneen was one of a dozen or so Americans enrolled at the time. The Irish were constrained from attending Trinity by the Catholic Church. John Charles McQuaid, the Archbishop of Dublin, threatened Irish attendees with the possibility of excommunication. This edict was reinforced regularly by the local clergy at Sunday Mass. Finally realizing the public relations aspect of consigning a significant number of young Irish students to hell's eternal fire and appreciative of the Church's budding ecumenical bent, the ban was lifted in 1970.

A majority of the students at Trinity, including Tom, lived on campus. Tom lived in Botany Bay, the dwelling which once housed Oscar Wilde. As part of the original construction, the buildings lacked many modern amenities. The rooms were notoriously cold and drafty during the winter months. Each "suite" had a small kitchen area, a living room with a small fireplace, and usually two bedrooms. Heat was derived solely from the fireplace. Tom and his roommate had a "man" who would clean on a regular basis and prepare the evening fire. On a few occasions, he invited me to join him for supper. Students, clothed in black gowns, dined in a large refectory, one of the original buildings. The protocol and traditions of centuries past, including Grace before meals, were still observed. The food, however, was consistently terrible.

THE DANDY

The prototypical Trinity man, at least in my mind's eye, was often seen strolling with other kindred spirits along Grafton Street, discussing, I presumed, some obscure Platonian tract. Although well put out, his garb was more distinct than distinguished: a tweed jacket, reinforced with leather at the elbows; a tie jauntily knotted over an acceptably wrinkled linen shirt; with a scarf - a confluence of color or perhaps Trinity blue - casually thrown over the shoulder. If a suit were the attire of the day, it would often be accompanied by a black lacquered, gold-capped cane. An unbuttoned raincoat loosely belted at the waist, even on fine days, was often part of the look.

The Trinity man would drink and consort at only the better places in town: Baileys and Davey Byrnes (where in James Joyce's *Ulysses* Leopold Bloom famously took his lunch - a gorgonzola cheese sandwich and a glass of Burgundy) were two favored bistros. His was a terribly sophisticated British accent, or at least, a terribly affected Irish one. Money seemed of little concern, and when he was noted in the back bar of Davy Byrnes, setting aside his martini to offer a stunningly attractive woman a cigarette from his gold cigarette case, it seemed altogether too elegant. It can also be said that some of the wildest parties in Dublin were given by Trinity-types, especially after rowing and rugby events.

Colleges were not the only institutions from which a medical license could be obtained. Apothecaries Hall was created back in the 1700s, at a time when pharmacists also rendered medical care. This being the case, it was felt they should also receive some formal medical training. "Pots Hall" remained in existence until 1970. During my time in Dublin, classroom instruction was not offered, and the institution acted only as an examining body. The "Pots" students acquired medical education on their own but had access to hospitals for the clinical work. Apothecaries Hall had established relationships with professors at UCD and Surgeons who would write the exams, conduct orals, and grade the candidates' efforts. Often, the students had begun their medical careers at other institutions and for whatever reason, usually academic, had dropped out. Many long-term, "chronic" students took the "Pots" route. The license allowed one to practice as a pharmacist or physician, but only in Ireland and England. The avenue of last resort for those wishing to obtain a medical license, it was the butt of some ridicule amongst students in the more established medical programs.

T he first half of my preregistration year passed rapidly. I enjoyed the college, the digs worked out well, and friends had been made. Science courses continued to be a challenge, as evidenced by my flunking Chemistry just before Christmas. Although not highly ranked in the hierarchy of difficult exams, a failure in the spring repeat would cancel any chance of getting home for the summer. And if I wasn't successful in the mid-August final try, I could be dropped from the program. So when classes resumed after the holidays there was certain to be considerable pressure to get the damn thing out of the way – a situation which left me a little depressed. Pat O'Brien, very kindly, invited me to his home in England for a few days prior to the holiday.

Pat's parents were great. His father, a doctor, as mentioned previously, had a very busy general practice in Gateshead. A handsome man, gregarious and socially adept, he would not be mistaken for anything other than Irish. High facial color may have indicated a fondness for the "drop," but it didn't deter him from maintaining a fine home and medical practice. Pat's mother was a very pleasant lady, especially nice to me, and an excellent cook. On occasion, I surmised she had her moments with her Irish boyo, but they seemed to get along well. Their conversation was a comfortable interplay between a husband and wife who had seen a lot of water flow under the bridge, but who'd managed to get through it all with their sense of humor intact. And as Pat noted, they still became a bit coquettish whenever the waltz, "Three O'clock in the Morning," was played. The whole scene was one with which I was not familiar.

My first Christmas in Dublin was spent with Tom Conneen at Trinity. His roommate, an Englishman, went home for the holidays. I had promptly accepted the invite as Miss Halligan had also left - to spend time with her family - and had closed the digs.

On Christmas Eve, Tom and I had drinks at the Metropole bar on O'Connell Street. A conversation was maintained with a young lady seated next to us, while she waited for her parents to arrive for dinner. The chat continued until her mother and father arrived, at which time they retired to a nearby table. Tom and I remained at the bar and continued talking until Tom interrupted.

"Gene. I think she likes you."

I returned a blank stare.

"So," he continued, "why don't you go over and see if you can get her to invite us for dinner tomorrow."

Dumbfounded, I replied, "You can't simply insert yourself into a family's Christmas!"

"Unless someone feeds us," Tom responded, "we're not going to eat. There's no food at my place and every restaurant will be closed."

His logic eventually won the day. Hesitantly, I approached their table, initiated a chat with the young lady, who in turn, introduced me to her parents. Details of the conversation are lost but somehow I implied that we would love to join them for Christmas dinner. Unbelievably, they said they would be delighted; so the following day, join them we did, along with assorted family members. A great time was had and the family appeared genuinely pleased to share their holiday with us. However, the unmitigated gall that we exhibited makes me cringe, even now, as I recount the story these decades later.

So ended 1955, a significant year for me. Twelve months earlier, I could not have imagined the changes which would take place in my life... Also, about that time, I received a letter from one of the wait-listed schools, the New York Medical College, offering me a place in their spring program. After much back and forth correspondence with Aunt Bertha, it was decided that I would stay put, with tuition costs being the major consideration.

1956 AND THE IRISH ECONOMY

Economically, during the 50s and for some time prior, Ireland was doing poorly. Employment at any level - menial to business and professional - was unavailable for much of the population. In Dublin, but more obviously in the country, the elderly and those of school age remained well represented while those in the twenty to fifty year age bracket were not seen in any significant concentration. Young people, including graduates of the country's universities and colleges, were forced to seek employment elsewhere – either in England or, more permanently, in the U.S. or Australia.

However, the dismal Irish economy served me well. The exchange rate, vis-a-vis, the American dollar, was seven shillings to one dollar. Ten dollars translated to three pounds and ten shillings. The following is offered for perspective: wages for mid-range workers - office staff, police, teachers - were between ten to fifteen pounds a week: thirty to forty-five dollars; men cut peat in the bogs, by hand, for approximately one pound per day: three to four dollars.

My board was less than ten dollars a week. Tuition at Surgeons was roughly one thousand dollars a year. In American money: seventeen cents bought a pint of Guiness; admission to a regular dance cost forty cents, while a more upscale venue charged eighty; cigarettes were twenty cents for a pack of ten. On a Saturday night, ten shillings - one dollar and fifty cents - allowed up to five pints of stout, a pack of cigarettes, admission to a dance, and change in my pocket at the end of the evening. The circumstances that placed me in Ireland during those years were providential; I could not have made it otherwise.

THE NEW YEAR

The core clientele in the digs remained stable at the start of the New Year: Dan Savage, the postman; Frank Gillan, the principal; Lorna, the spinster lady; and Joe, Miss Halligan's nephew - all in residence for many years. By this point, the initial forced cordiality I had experienced was no longer. That threshold having been crossed, I was now officially a member of the group. It was insisted, for instance, that I join the regulars for a New Year's Eve drink in the upstairs parlor, an invite which sealed the deal as to my new status.

Newcomers included two gentlemen from UCD: Ray Mc-Loughlin and Jim Orange. Ray, from Ballinasloe, County Galway, was a brilliant student in the engineering program, who also played Rugby and put the shot in field events for the College. (After graduation he enjoyed an outstanding business career, and at one point, captained Ireland's national rugby team.)

That Jim Orange possessed the qualities one finds in an outstanding lawyer - argumentative, articulate, confrontational and intelligent – was evident to everyone in the house, long before he received his degree.

(He subsequently established a law practice – presently one of Dublin's most prestigious - which he still maintains. On a recent trip to Dublin we met briefly. Other than a hint of mellowness and a minimally altered physical appearance, Jim was as remembered - with all the aforementioned qualities firmly in place.)

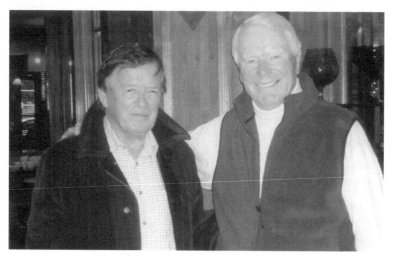
Gene and Jim Orange - 2011 Alumni Visit

My goals for the up-coming year were modest: pass my ex-ams (including the Chemistry repeat), and hopefully go home for the summer. It had been awhile since I trod my home turf. To paraphrase Tom Jones, singing in his fine Welch baritone, it's good to touch the green, green grass of home.

As with any rooming house, occupancy was always in flux. Residents stayed a night, others for weeks or months. Whatever the length of stay, all were informed of the house rules by Miss Halligan. That this decree was not merely a suggestion, but enforced, was illustrated on one occasion.

Adelaide O'Hagan was an attractive young woman, entered in the physiotherapy program at UCD. She joined our household sometime in late March, with plans to stay until her exam in the spring. Her room was next to mine on the second floor. One evening she mentioned an exam was upcoming, and as preparation, asked if I could make my body available as a study aid for the identification of various muscle groups.

"Yes," I quickly responded. "Anything to help." In truth, I feared her disappointment, for even on a good day, my un-ripped torso could not be described as anything but scrawny.

Not worrying too much, one afternoon we met in her room. My shirt off, I stretched out on her bed, face down. Adelaide sat beside me and slowly moved her hands over my back. After a few minutes of this increasingly pleasant activity, we were interrupted by a hard knock on the door, which then quickly opened.

There stood Miss Halligan. "There'll be none of that in this house," she said.

"But...," I began.

"There's no buts about it," she replied. "And as for you, young lady, I'll speak with you later."

Adelaide stood there as if dumbstruck. Sheepishly, I put on my shirt and went to my room. How Miss Halligan became aware of our benign tryst was a puzzle, as she was situated two floors below and we were very quiet. Adelaide left the digs shortly afterward, and my only regret was that I hadn't been able to contribute, in a more meaningful way, to her exam success.

In the spring of 1956, Dr. O'Brien arranged for Pat and me to attend the Grand National Steeplechase at Aintree in England with him. The race had a long tradition in England, but my knowledge derived solely from the film, *National Velvet*, starring Elizabeth Taylor and Mickey Rooney. Knowledgeable of the history or not, one could not help getting caught up in the carnival-like atmosphere of the event, fueled by the buzz of anticipation rippling through the crowd. Visible among the more affluent in the stands behind us, were ladies bedecked in gowns and imposing millinery creations; beside them, men in tuxedos and top hats leaned casually on walking sticks, their other hand holding the obligatory champagne flute.

Considered the most grueling of steeple chase events, the course stretched over seven miles with thirty fences, including water jumps. Stands were available, but the majority viewed the event at ground level. Unless equipped with binoculars, the only close-up view of the horses was on one of their two circuits by the main enclosure. However, the commentary supplied through loud speakers, coupled with the energy and enthusiasm of the spectators, conjured up adequate imagery.

This particular day achieved an unfortunate distinction. Devon Loch, the Queen Mother's horse, ridden by Dick Francis, had cleared all 30 fences, and with 50 yards left to the finish and a four length lead, stumbled, fell, and lost the race. A dead silence prevailed in the crowd. The winning horse and jockey received only faint applause. It has remained one of the greatest misadventures in Grand National history. Dick Francis, following his riding career, went on to achieve considerable fame as one of England's most popular and prolific mystery writers. The phrase, "to do a Devon Loch," has since become a euphemism for snatching defeat from the jaws of victory.

Dan Savage, a resident whom I enjoyed immensely, had been with Miss Halligan a number of years. A letter carrier, working out of the General Post Office in Dublin, he had left his home in Galway some twelve years earlier. With black hair, sallow complexion, deep-set eyes and shallow cheeks, there was the brush of the Spaniard about him.

"Could be," he said. "The west is full of us black Irish. Lots of randy sailors on those Spanish traders back then."

Dan's social life, like the rest of us, consisted of a few pints on Saturday nights and the occasional party. When one made twelve pounds a week, with three pounds for board, not much was left for the finer things. Occasionally Dan and I headed out together. As were many Irishmen, Dan was well-versed in the stories, poems, and history of his country. And, of course, he loved to sing.

Pubs which allowed singing and recitation were Dan's choices, and although not my preference, Dan insisted I come along. "It's great craic," he guaranteed, and he was right. A place off Camden Street and another in the Harold's Cross section of Dublin were his particular favorites, most remembered on winter nights as being wonderfully warm. A dozen or so tables were scattered about the lounge with stand-up counters along the walls; a small area was cleared for the musicians. After the crowd had settled in, patrons, in their turn, stood up, told a story, recited a poem, or more usually, sang a song.

The Irish, it seems, are at ease with melancholy, comfortable with brooding clouds and grayness, suspicious of sunny times. To quote W.B. Yeats: "They have an abiding sense of tragedy which sustains them through temporary periods of joy." The songs and readings were somber fare: dealing with the "troubles," the 1916 uprising and its martyrs, the Diaspora of the

1840's - all done with great emotion. "Kevin Barry" ("just a lad of eighteen summers," and a medical student at UCD, executed by the British for his part in the 1916 uprising), and "The Rising of the Moon" were among those songs I remember. No McNamara's Band here. The playwright, Brendan Behan, occasionally in attendance, always contributed, and in Gaelic.

Dan's favorite vocal rendition, "Come Back Paddy Reilly," written by Percy French – although a reference to emigration – had a more lighthearted bent. With pint raised and eyes closed, he'd sing the ballad in his fine baritone voice, encouraging all to join in the chorus.

Shouts of approval followed. "Fine man, Dan..." "Ah, grand it is..." Courtesy was extended to the presenter and one didn't boo or clap during the recital. Unless invited, no one sang along. Dan, although a relatively young man, had false teeth. Often he found it difficult to synchronize lips, words, and plate, especially after a pint or two. So there were occasional pauses during his rendering which allowed his dental appliance to slip into place.

"The Four Farrellys" was his trademark poem. Also written by Percy French, it told the story of an Irishman, who having checked into a London hotel one evening, noticed the name of a Francis Farrelly on the register. Later that night, over a drink, the man wondered which Farrelly this might be and began a recollection of the Francis Farrelly's of his acquaintance in Ireland. Was it the papist he knew from the North? The rebel from the South? His college mate in the East? Or perhaps a young man he was acquainted with from the West? The appropriate rendition of the poem required the ability to mimic the accent of each region. Dan did this to perfection.

Dan recited the verses that described the Francis of the North, South and East in his usual impressive fashion. But on every occasion, when he reached the final verse, describing the young man from the West, where Dan was from, his demeanor changed and his voice softened.

"Or were you that Francis Farrelly I met so long ago?
In the bog below Belmulett, in the county of Mayo?
That long-legged, freckled Frances with the deep-set, wistful eyes,
That seemed to take their color from those ever-changing skies.
That put his flute together as I sketched the distant scene,
And played me "Planxy Kelly" and the "Wakes of Inniskeen,"
That told me in the Autumn he'd be Bailin' to the West
To try and make his fortune and send money to the rest.
And would I draw a picture of the place where he was born,
And he'd hang it up, and look at it, and not feel so forlorn,
And when I had it finished, you got up from where you sat,
And you said, "Well, you're the Divil, and I can't say more than that."

(About here Dan's voice broke, eyes filled and tears soon followed.)

"Oh' if you're that Francis Farrelly, your fortune may be small,
But I'm thinking- thinking- Francis, that I love you best of all;
And I never can forget you- though it's years and years ago-
In the bog below Belmullet, in the County of Mayo."

Once finished, Dan raised his pint and acknowledged the applause. After he sat down and composed himself, his usual comment was something along the lines of "Jasus, ain't this a terrible bollocks of a country?"

During these months Dan Savage acquired a lady friend. She had recently moved from her home in Galway and taken a position at Clery's department store in downtown Dublin. They apparently had been seeing each other for a few weeks prior to Dan presenting her to our group at tea one evening. Tall, well put together, with a quiet demeanor, she was welcomed, inspected, and accepted as worthy of our Dan. Frank Gillan was especially gracious with nothing untoward to say about the lady - even after she left.

The dating continued in fits and starts through the spring. Dan confided he didn't want to rush things, needed to think things through. "Sure, there's plenty of time," he said. Dan was at least forty years old; she looked considerably younger.

Dan's interest was piqued when she began doing his laundry. The previous desultory conversations regarding his intentions, their compatibility or future plans, were now more animated; the notion that a corner had been turned in their relationship was almost palpable.

Dan admitted as much to me one evening in the sitting room. "Ah, she's a grand girl, Gene. And it's only recently I've come to notice."

"Yes," I replied, "a fine looking woman."

"You know," Dan continued, "I've really started to give it some thought."

"About what, Dan?"

"A token, a ring maybe, to show my interest. Nothing serious," he added. "Just something, you know, to keep it going like it is, ease the conscience a bit."

"Sounds like a start," I said.

"And one day..." He paused. "You never know..."

On he went, illustrating similarities: their Galway origins, how both were devout Catholics, each into song and poetry, the shared loss of a parent at an early age. But somehow the overture, though beguiling, seemed but a cover. Something was missing.

Then, just before we headed into tea, Dan leaned toward me, his tone more confidential. "Gene, you should see how she does my laundry. Pure white they are, the underwear, the stains gone; the shirts, not a wrinkle, and starched!"

I knew it, I thought. *Now we have it.*

"And, to top it off," he continued, "she doesn't get mad when I get bollixed drunk once in a while."

"Dan," I replied, "looks like all the essentials are in place."

This conversation with Dan illustrated a dictum not initially appreciated, but increasingly apparent: that every "true" tale was often a mix of fanciful illusion and feigned artlessness. A verbal sleight-of-hand was employed, not necessarily meant to betray; for just as a card shark is expected to cheat, so too, the storyteller was expected to obscure authenticity with a clutter of irrelevant asides. The listener was forced to chip away at the facade until some semblance of fact emerged; although often at the completion of the chat, one knew nothing more than at its inception. In relaxed settings, maintaining these exchanges for extended periods of time (often without the hint of a smile), was, and is, a uniquely Irish talent.

A Song and Story Man

As Percy French has been mentioned on a couple of occasions, it would be appropriate to note the background of one of Ireland's greatest songwriters and entertainers. His considerable talents included watercolor painting and writing plays, short stories, and verse. In his day (late 1800s), he took on the trappings of the bard - the ancient Irish storyteller, who in a simple style spoke of the mundane and commonplace in life, but with a facility and wit that transcended generations and social class.

Percy loitered through Trinity long enough to develop his musical and artistic talents, and to obtain a degree in Civil Engineering (at his father's insistence; Percy preferred the Classics). The variety of his subsequent job postings provided much of the material for his later literary efforts.

On a trip to Dublin for an alumni gathering some years ago, I took a walk along the Grand Canal. Stopping at a bench to watch the ducks and debris float by, I noticed a metal plaque affixed to its back. It read: "In memory of William Percy French, 1854-1920." Beneath was his epitaph:

> **"Remember me is all I ask, and yet,**
> **If the memory proves a task – forget."**

That same day I went to a Dublin book store - Hodges Figgis - and asked the clerk, a young man, if they carried anything by Mr. French. He had never heard of him, and the older man he referred me to had only a dim recollection of the name and added, "We certainly have nothing of his in stock." He suggested an antique book shop on Dawson Street. As I made my way through town, I thought, Whoever said that *"life is short and fame is fleeting,"* was right on the money.

Home for the Summer

The second half of the preregistration year had gone well. The previously failed Chemistry exam succumbed to concentrated effort and was easily passed as were the other finals for the year. Social and study routines were pretty much established and I had become more comfortable in the situation I found myself. The additional year I was required to take, which I had been upset about, was over. If everything worked out in the end, I rationalized, it would have been a small penalty.

I wasn't sure how I'd spend my time before the semester started, but as usual, Bertha's brief letter provided direction.

Dear Gene,

Think we need to get you home for the summer and see what you look like. Check with American Express – see what ships are sailing and when, and I'll get a check to you. Nothing fancy, please...

Accordingly, I boarded a ship at Cobh, more tramp steamer than liner, whose itinerary originated in Algiers. After a stop to pick up cargo and passengers at Cadiz, Spain, it had made its way to Ireland. There were no more than one hundred passengers aboard, half of whom were workers on their way to jobs in the United States. The food was good and my cabin surprisingly large, but amenities were lacking. A small bar was open for a few hours each night, and other than a worn jukebox, playing unfamiliar music, no entertainment was offered. An engine malfunction required overnight repairs in Halifax, Nova Scotia. Two days later we disembarked at the port of New York, my first foothold on U.S. soil in a year and a half. I was glad to be home, if for no other reason, than to replenish a wardrobe virtually unchanged since my departure.

My father was pleased with my progress, as was Aunt Bertha, although her comments were more tempered, such as: "Well, at least it's a step in the right direction."

My mother, whom I visited a few days later, seemingly had only one concern: "Are you sure you won't be staying there when you finish?" I assured her this wouldn't be the case. As my mother, she said, she always wanted me nearby. A heartfelt, though ironic, sentiment such as this was brushed aside, not remotely considered an expression of her affection for me. Her absence over the years, coupled with the bias in my father's family, resulted in her being a secondary presence in my life. As had been her custom for years, she rented a cottage nearby at Point Judith for a week during the summer. I seldom visited, the usual excuse: my long work day.

The summer passed quickly. The Co-Op took me back, and as expected, the stink, the endless stream of fish and a dull knife were as before. Fridays at the Country Club provided spending money for the week. If it happened to rain, curtailing golf for the day, it made for a threadbare few days. Again, the only social respite was the occasional country and western dance.

By summer's end I had made enough money to fund my passage back to Ireland and provide part of the tuition for a year at Surgeons. A mid-September departure from New York was booked on the *RMS Mauretania*.

In the summer of 1956, the great transatlantic ships could still be seen along the piers of New York's North River. The Queens (*Mary* and *Elizabeth*), the *SS France*, and the *United States*, still plied their elegant trade. But change was in the air: jet aircraft had arrived, and a trip that took days by sea was now accomplished in hours. Little did I know when I boarded the *Mauretania* that September day in 1956, that journeys such as mine were the tail end, the final curtain call for an era and a life style.

A Transatlantic Crossing

A ft of the great liner, New York's North River shimmered in the heat of an Indian summer afternoon. The tugboats had taken their positions. Piercing the sweep of the massive hull, gangplanks were lined with boarding passengers while on the docks below, longshoreman, stripped to their waists, loaded the last of the pallets. High above the curve of the hull two smokestacks trickled white exhaust into a blue sky.

Tentatively I made my way up a swaying rope bridge to an entryway high above the water line. The sun, reflecting off the steel, blinded; my ears rang with the screech of hoists as they swung past. There was a chill, a shiver of apprehension as I stepped into the coolness of the *RMS Mauritania*.

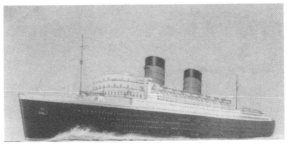

RMS Mauritania

Along corridors lined with luggage, I made my way. The air was fragrant with the smell of cigars and leather, and as ladies passed, the trail of their perfumes. A descent of four levels brought me to D deck, absent the affluent aromas of the upper reaches, where I found my cabin. The door was ajar. After a knock, I pushed it open. Inside were two men, one leaning against the wash basin haloed by its light, the other seated on the lower bunk, elbows on his knees, with a drink cradled between his hands.

"Sorry," I said, "I'll come back later."

The man on the bunk beckoned, "Come on in, me boyo, just a friend seeing me off."

Then he stood, a big man whose frame filled the cabin. His suit was gray with a tie loosely knotted beneath an unbuttoned, detachable collar. His cap, pulled low over his forehead, shadowed his face. As he turned, his profile, reflected in the mirror, appeared disjointed. For a moment, I thought the mirror was cracked.

The man reached for a bottle, tilted in the sink. "Join us?"

"No thanks," I replied. "I'm going to watch us shove off. I'll see you later."

The tugs had nudged the liner from its berth and headed it slowly upstream into the river traffic. The New York skyline emerged, the line of skyscrapers bathed in a fluorescent dusk. The Statue of Liberty at the harbor entrance, shadowed in the early evening, moved me, as I imagined it did for all who looked upon it for the first time. Soon the pilot boat was a small speck bobbing its way back to the harbor through the mist. As the shoreline slowly receded, gusts of brisk ocean breeze thinned the ranks of those remaining on the foredeck; soon the ship settled into the rhythmic lift and fall of the Atlantic rollers. New York was just a smudge of gray as I headed back to the cabin.

The man was sitting on the edge of the lower bunk staring at the floor, fingers dangling, with a glass wedged between his heels.

"Hello, again. I'm Gene, Gene McKee."

"Seamus Dorcan here," the man said and extended his hand. Face on, I understood the reflection in the mirror. Although the brim of his cap was pulled down, it couldn't conceal the fixed stare of his left eye. Beneath it, a flesh colored device was plugged into his cheek, apparently attached to underlining structures, but without any resemblance to the adjacent facial color or contour.

"Not too pretty, eh?" Seamus said. His half smile stretched

the edges of a scar which extended from the side of his nose to his left ear, where it sharply turned to follow the line of his jaw. An opaque blue eye showed no movement. The effect, even in partial light, was grotesque, like a Halloween mask that didn't quite fit.

"Sorry about staring," I said. "It just took me by surprise."

"Can hardly stand it myself," Seamus replied, as he dabbed at the trickle from his nose.

"So enough about me," he continued, "let's hear about you." Seamus retrieved the bottle from the sink and poured himself a drink. "Join me?" I shook my head no. "So you're off to Ireland are you, me young friend? And how old might you be?"

"Twenty-one," I replied, "twenty-two in a few months."

Seamus placed a pillow behind his back and settled into the lower bunk. "And what," he asked, "would be the reason for this grand adventure?"

While Seamus sipped, I briefly spoke of the difficulties I had encountered gaining acceptance to an American medical school, and as a last resort, having applied to and been accepted at a school in Ireland.

"I finished a preliminary year in June, so this will be my first go in the medical school," I told him. "Not crazy about the whole idea; it's more to please the family... Anyway," I added, "if I don't make it, I still have the military, and I'm fine with that."

Other than an occasional grunt there was only silence from the figure stretched out on the bunk before me. Carefully, I reached over and turned on the light over the bunk. Seamus had fallen asleep, his head propped against the wall of the cabin; spit had dripped onto his lapel and his cheek was smeared with a trickle from his nose. This, I thought, was going to be one helluva trip.

I saw little of my roommate over the next three days. Coming in late I found him asleep, usually still dressed, with an empty glass on the floor beside his bunk. A green scapular dangled from the springs above. In the morning when I awoke, he was gone and most days could be found, no matter the weather, stretched out on a deckchair, wrapped in a blanket. Trays of food left by the door remained untouched, and except for a diminishing box of Schrafft's chocolates with a "Bon Voyage, Surgical Three" card attached, the man apparently did not eat.

This was my first trip on a true ocean liner. Why the *Mauretania* was chosen for this voyage, I don't remember; probably because it was the least expensive option. This ship, I learned, was the second *Mauretania*; the original, a sister ship of the *Lusitania*, had owned the speed record for Atlantic crossings in its day but was now consigned to the scrap heap.

One of the Cunard liners, the *Mauretania* was smaller than the Queens, but otherwise British in every detail. There were three distinct classes and, typically, n'er the twain did meet. I, obviously, was in the third-class section, well below the water line, in the aft portion of the ship. The rooms were small to the extent that two people could not dress at the same time. There were bunk beds, a small sink, and a closet which accommodated very little. Common toilets and bath facilities were situated at intervals along the corridor. The meals, however, were outstanding, with multiple courses. There was afternoon tea and snacks and desserts available before you headed to your stateroom for the night. One could not complain about the variety or quantity of the food.

The second-class section, clearly demarcated, occupied the center of the ship. This, I was told, was the province of honeymooners and middle class, older couples. First-class passengers occupied the forward portion of the ship, so as not to be downward of the smokestacks belching smoke and soot.

One of the advantages of being young, single, and male on the ships of that time was the opportunity to socialize with the daughters of first-class passengers. An invitation/summons was extended to me and two others in my age group, to present ourselves at a specific time, in the first-class lounge. Suitably dressed in shirt, tie, and jacket, we were escorted by a ship's officer to our appointment. The impressions remain: carpeted corridors bordered by dark wood wainscoting; staterooms whose ornate wooden doors muffled voices and sprigs of laughter from within; the fragrance of cigars. The first-class lounge was semi-circular in shape with two large mirrors over the bar and ships lanterns hanging on either side. Hundreds of bottles lined the glass shelves. An Oriental rug filled the center of the floor. Large windows on either side of the lounge gave an unobstructed view of the ocean hundreds of feet below.

On the occasions I was in attendance, twice on this trip, everyone was formally dressed for dinner: the men, handsome in tuxedos, and gowned ladies perfectly coiffed. Everyone seemed terribly sophisticated with their cocktails and cigarettes. We young men chatted briefly with the parents then socialized with the young ladies until dinner. A section of the floor without carpet allowed dancing, with the music supplied by a formally attired quartet. We dined apart from the adults and I distinctly remember my first taste of champagne. The young ladies wanted to visit third-class after dinner, where the lounges were livelier and less formal. With parental permission, some did and they always enjoyed themselves.

Also aboard was a contingent of about ten girls from New Zealand traveling to England. I, along with my two third-class companions, partied our way, pretty much non-stop, across the Atlantic with them. A large amount of money was spent on alcohol - champagne became our drink of choice - but even now I consider it money well spent.

The younger generation of ships officers, also hot on the trail of single ladies, was quite successful. They employed a very creative stratagem. After they obtained the names of the more attractive women on board, they would wait until the second or third night and then invite them to a party in the officers' mess.

Of course, any young girl's head would be turned by the opportunity to share conversation and cocktails with a handsome, young officer in his gleaming whites. A significant number of women were removed from the availability pot as a result of this underhanded maneuver.

An Atlantic storm cleared the decks one afternoon, and as I passed through the lounge I saw Seamus, by himself, at a corner table. Tea was being served, as was the mid-afternoon custom, with music provided by a pianist and a violinist valiantly attempting to maintain his balance in the heavy seas.

"Mind if I join you?" I asked.

"Sit down, me friend," he replied. Seamus hadn't shaved and the gray stubble of one cheek was a stark contrast to the shine from the pink rubber surface of the other. "Sure, we haven't seen much of each other this trip," said Seamus, as he raised his glass. "And why not, me boyo?" he continued. "Enjoy yourself. These are great days for ya, though you may not think it now."

A waiter brought me tea and a plate of crackers. We chatted as the wind howled and the ship lifted and fell through the angry sea. Soon the violinist and the pianist packed up and the lounge cleared, save for a waiter who was clearing tables.

"Tell me, Seamus, where were you in America?"

"A famous hospital, in Minnesota."

"The Mayo Clinic?" I asked.

"The very place. And there it was that the bastards took away half me face. Some kind of cancer, they said, with a fancy name, spread into my eye, it did." He paused. "If I had known what I was to go through, I would never have left Cloghan."

"But Seamus," I said, "you'd have died for sure. And now look at the years still ahead for you."

"Aye, Gene, but there's some things in life worse than dying, when death would be a blessing." He grabbed his glass as it started to slide off the table, finished its contents, grimacing as he swallowed, then called to the waiter for another.

"Tell me, Seamus, are you in much pain? Looks like it's hard for you to swallow."

"Sure the pain's constant but it's the throat that's the worst part, burned raw with the poison that trickles down. It's only the drink that makes it bearable." Seamus paused. "But that will pass one day, and I suppose I'll get used to shaving half a face and seeing the shudder of strangers. It's tomorrow when we walk down that gang-plank that starts the real ordeal. Two months ago, Gene, I left Ireland a fine robust man, if I say so myself, and now look at me, one of Damien's own."

"People understand, Seamus."

"No, me boyo, not the Irish. The cruelest people in the world they are, especially to their own. I can hear them now, wailing for me poor wife with her terrible cross to bear, my daughter taunted in school. And then, of course, the good Father, with his palaver about God's grace and sharing the pain of Jesus, all that pious bullshit. Och, I can't stand the thought of it all."

Seamus sat back in his chair. "I tell you, me lad, I'd rather be dead. If it weren't for me ma, I'd get it over with. But she sold half the farm to pay those Yankee doctors and wouldn't it be selfish of me now, not to show off their handiwork?"

As the ship creaked and spray lashed the wide lounge windows, Seamus spoke of the family farm in Cloghan, which although mostly bog, had, in his mind, a beauty of its own. He recollected walks with his brothers at the end of the day, the land cloaked in the shadow of the evening, fields pocked with misty pools that stretched to the hills beyond. In the pub on Saturday nights there was always great "craic" and Seamus chuckled at the memory of two summers past when Offaly, his county, "destroyed altogether" Kerry in the Hurling Cup Final.

Of his wife he spoke little, but the remembrance of his twelve-year-old daughter, Moira ("a bonnie lass if there ever was one"), brought a smile to his face. "You should see her, Gene, eyes blue like china and blonde hair that falls half down her back. She'll be a beauty one day." Seamus shook his head. "What will she think when she sees her dad now? Anyway," he continued, "it is not just me, Gene; you've got to face the hard cut, yourself."

"Suppose you're right, Seamus," I replied. "Guess we're both wondering what we'll find on the other side of the gangplank."

The party, our last night aboard, ended just before the tender arrived to transport us to the dock in Cobh. As I headed back to the cabin, I passed Seamus, his face hooded, heading to the departure deck.

"Seamus, wait up and I'll go with you."

"No Gene, I'm heading on, but I've enjoyed your company. And if I don't see you again, the best of Irish luck to you." A small smile came to his face. "If there is such a thing. Anyway watch out for the girls and easy on the gargle and you'll be fine."

I watched as he made his way down the gangplank to one of the waiting boats, stopping once to adjust his cap.

A short time later I was aboard a crowded tender chugging its way through choppy waters to the pier at Cobh. In a semi-circle surrounding the harbor, multi-colored homes made an attractive back-drop. Standing tall, dominating the landscape, was the magnificent St. Coleman's Cathedral, perched on a hill behind the city. Of Gothic architecture, it was built in the early 1900s, the cost largely underwritten by American and Australian donations. Famous for its carillon, resonating at fifteen-minute intervals, it was the last sight of Ireland for millions of emigrants. Greeted (as if on cue), by the chimes of the cathedral, we made land-fall and joined the line for Customs.

I didn't see Seamus again until later, when I was seated on a bus in Cobh, waiting to be taken to the train station in Cork. For a moment, I thought he was alone, but then a young blond girl, wearing a blue dress, came into view, holding his hand. A woman, I assumed to be his wife, had an arm around Seamus's waist and as they passed, appeared to be crying.

Back in Dublin, Miss Halligan welcomed me back to the digs. Finally finished with the sciences, I looked forward to anatomy and physiology. Little could I have imagined the drudgery that awaited me over the next eighteen months. But, ignorance, as they say, is bliss.

FIRST MEDICAL YEAR

The College of Surgeons, at that time, employed the classical European paradigm for the education of physicians. The first year and a half, students dealt primarily with two subjects: anatomy and physiology. For most, the intense focus on anatomy had little application other than the discipline of memorization unless one was considering a surgical career.

A.K. Henry was the Professor of Anatomy. A world renowned anatomist, author of various texts in his field, he had fashioned a remarkable career – including serving as a surgeon in the French army during WWI, before assuming the Surgeon's position. Various honors had come his way over the years and it was something of a coup for the college to have him on their faculty.

Tall and very thin, the professor, garbed in a starched, loosely fitting white lab coat, presented his material in a scarcely inflected monotone - a sleep-inducing eddy of quiet noise. His face - pale skin stretched taut over bony angles - appeared shrink-wrapped. Bent over the podium, long cobbled fingers clasped beneath his chin, the image was of frailty. Clearly A.K., about seventy-years-old at the time, was on the sunset side of an illustrious career.

Cadavers were assigned for dissection in the Anatomy Theater. Dealing with a dead body for the first time – the pungent smell of preservatives, the leather-like skin, the fixed gaze – produced an initial uneasiness which rapidly resolved. Four students worked on the upper half of the body and four, the lower half. When the assigned half was completed, a new cadaver was obtained and the roles reversed. At any given time, eight-to-ten bodies were in various stages of dissection.

Along with three others, I was assigned a male cadaver. Over the ensuing weeks, directed by instructors, we explored and identified the anatomy of the pelvis and lower extremities. At a nearby table, four students, including a female student I'll call Ingrid, were similarly engaged in a dissection of the lower half of a female cadaver. Tall, attractive, with a decent figure, Ingrid presented as something of a "goody two shoes." Prim in dress, proper in demeanor, diligent in study, abstinent of cigarettes and alcohol, she offered an impressive facade of discipline and restraint. Her dissections, I noted, were accomplished wearing white gloves lest her hands be exposed to the formaldehyde-induced skin damage the rest of us endured.

A consensus was reached by our all-male group that it would be great fun to bring this paragon of propriety down a peg or two; all we needed was a ploy that would inflict the most embarrassment. The answer lay before us in the Anatomy Theater. Our assigned male cadaver was relatively young with well-defined musculature. But most impressive, in spite of his moribund status, was an extravagant genital apparatus – well-hung by any measure – and fairly firm to boot. Accordingly we named him Willie, after classmate Willie Hickey, who had something of a reputation as a lady's man. With this bounty before us, our perverted minds coalesced around a plan.

Early one morning we separated Willie from his male member and placed it between the thighs, at the vaginal intoitus, of Ingrid's cadaver. Clustered around our emasculated Willie, we awaited her arrival. Besides ourselves in anticipation, we imagined the possibilities: would she scream, possibly faint, perhaps cry?

Ingrid approached the cadaver and carefully put on her white gloves. We muffled our mirth as she leaned over for a closer look. Then, with Willie's wiener daintily held between two gloved fingers, she turned and faced us. In a voice that filled the room, she proclaimed, "Seems one of you lads left in a hurry last night." The assembly, most in on the prank, convulsed in laughter and applauded in appreciation of her classic rejoinder. And there we stood, the tables turned, blushing in embarrassment.

After the episode, we – the instigators – offered something of an apology and hoped she wasn't too upset. Her response surprised us: "I thought it was great fun; can't wait to tell my girlfriends back home."

On the positive side, the incident broke the ice somewhat and we all became quite friendly. In later conversations, Ingrid said she was well aware of the perception many had of her, but her feeling was "so be it." She was determined to avoid any distraction that might affect her ability to complete the program. With continued exam success and the probability of graduation quite certain, we noted significant modifications in the virtuous lifestyle of her earlier years.

As the dissection progressed, on-going testing was accomplished. One form of exam, the viva, tested a student's recall of recently completed dissections. Prior to the exam, instructors placed colored pins in, or attached ties to, a variety of muscles, blood vessels, nerves, etc. The students filed through, transcribed their answers, and handed them in as they exited the room. Exam results were skewed, however. Although instructors circulated in the room, the occasional student, bent on disruption, surreptitiously removed a pin or two which he inserted, haphazardly, into other locations on the cadaver. This created a different set of answers for those following and a problem for those grading the exercise. The culprit also faced a dilemma. Being the last student able to submit reasonable answers he became the prime suspect - so would he forfeit the exam to avoid detection?

Another educational modality, separate from the college curriculum, was the Grind. These were sessions conducted by instructors or senior students proficient in a particular subject who wished to make extra money. Grinds in anatomy were very popular, with Tom Gary, an older man and anatomy instructor at the College of Surgeons for years, the favorite choice. As the story was told to me, Tom first worked in the department in a menial capacity, but on his own developed an interest in and extensive knowledge of the subject. Befriended and encouraged by A.K. Henry, the Anatomy professor, Tom's expertise became such that he was formally recognized with the title of Tutor and Prosector in Anatomy. A quiet man, seemingly devoid of social life, Tom's world revolved around his work at the college and the satisfaction derived, along with a few shillings, from the Grinds.

Charging half a crown (35 cents) per student, he convened sessions at his small apartment on Duke Street. In the front room, a large wooden box was filled with bones, some burnished to a bright sheen from use over the years. Once the area for discussion had been agreed upon, Tom rummaged through the box, selected the applicable bones and the Grind began. Students sat around a round, wooden table, illumined by a single overhead light. Tom's anatomic knowledge was encyclopedic and usually he possessed the patience of Job. (However, when his exasperation achieved critical mass he was known to dismiss the whole group until they exhibited evidence of prior study.)

What set Tom apart was his attempt to make anatomy, the driest of subjects, both interesting and logical. Common sense, he insisted, explained why every protuberance, depression, curve or articulation on a bone had to be exactly where it was, for that portion of the skeleton to function properly.

A typical session might start: "Good evening, gentlemen. Tonight we discuss the carpals, the bony structures that comprise the wrist. Very important, as they stabilize the entire upper arm..." In considerable detail, Tom would discuss the two rows of dense, irregularly shaped bones and their soft tissue attachments, with some reference to proximate blood vessel and nerve distribution. "But, most important," he'd add, "you must be able to quickly recall their names and in the correct order (frequently a question in the orals). Tom had a flair for the inventive mnemonic, and such was the case in this instance when he offered the following: Some Lovers Try Positions That They Cannot Handle - Scaphoid, Lunate, Triquetrum, Pisiform, Trapezium, Trapezoid, Capitate, Hamate." Imagination piqued, the memory jog prompted the immediate recall of the eight bones in question. The sessions lasted an hour and everyone participated. Before we were dismissed, Tom would go around the table with a question or two for each of us pertinent to the evening's discussion.

Tom was an outstanding resource for hundreds of students who labored through anatomy over the years. (On a recent visit to Surgeons, I noticed his picture on a wall in the small lecture room adjoining the Anatomy Theater and later learned that a research fund in anatomy had been set up in his name. It was nice to know he had not been forgotten.)

Most social activities occurred on Friday and Saturday nights. During the first medical year, Pat O'Brien was either in the digs or living close by, so we'd head out together. The first priority was to ensure adequate funding. If the coffers were low, Miss Halligan, if in a good mood, usually came through with ten shillings or occasionally a pound note.

McGrath's pub was our first stop. The proprietor, Joe Mc-Grath, was a big-boned, solid yolk of a man with a thatch of black hair. His pugnacious appearance, accentuated by a prominent jaw, became, when he smiled, modestly cherubic. His was a working man's pub with only the occasional UCD student in evidence. Trinity types were an unknown species.

McGrath's served a good pint and offered a popular bar game: Skittles. Played on a table with a sloped surface, the object of the game was to sink a ball into a series of pockets of varying difficulty, without overturning the skittles (small wooden pins) fronting them. The game was usually played with a partner, and if you continued to win, you "owned" the table; challenges were accepted from the list of those signed up to play. Jack Nugent and Frank O'Reilly come to mind as being one of the better teams.

A more practical reason for our allegiance to Joe: he allowed Pat and me "quiet tick." This accommodation allowed us to charge drinks, which were paid for at a later time - a privilege few had, especially students. Why Joe trusted us is unclear although our debt was always paid, if not always on time. Even more extraordinary were the times when, after a couple of pints, we borrowed money from the bar so we could continue the night at another establishment. Joe knew full well that was our plan but still complied in most instances.

The Toby Jug

After McGrath's, the next destination was the Toby Jug pub, the Surgeons hangout, located near the Gaiety Theatre on King Street. Frank Swift was the proprietor, Simon his assistant. The lounge was small and on Friday or Saturday nights, filled to capacity. The clientele were students, mostly male. Occasionally an unsuspecting soul brought his date into the horny assemblage. If he remained by her side for the duration of the evening, all would be fine, but if he as much as availed himself of the men's room, the odds of getting anywhere near the young lady for the remainder of the night were slim to none.

At some point during the evening there was an eruption of song, offering little resemblance to the original work. The repertoire ranged from "Galway Bay" and "Glasgow Town" to "Old Man River." Frank's pleas to "Keep it down, boys!" merited barely a glance. As the clock inched toward closing, Frank began the chant: "Now time, gentlemen, now time." His face, florid to start, became crimson, beads of sweat gathered on his forehead, and veins distended above a tight white collar. Initially pleading, he soon became exasperated. "For Jasus sake, get the feck out of here!" Eventually we did, with the night still young.

The best place to meet women was at a dance. A local favorite, the "Arts Hop," convened Friday nights at a small hall on Baggot Street, just down from the Shelburne Hotel. It featured Humphrey Murphy and his trio playing their signature tune: the "Wood Choppers Ball." Admittance was half a crown; if not available, the iron fence at the adjacent Huguenot Cemetery, once scaled, provided an alternative means of entry. The crowd was composed primarily of students, the majority from UCD, and girls who worked locally. Awash in stout, disheveled, and reeking of cigarettes, we presented an impressively unattractive package to the fair maidens in attendance. And then we wondered why we usually walked home alone.

The Four Provinces, nearby on Harcourt Street, also a popular dance destination, was favored by students of color. White males were frequently in the minority. The "Four P's" had a reputation, probably unjustified, as a place where "loose" women went to meet "black" students - "black" defined as anyone who wasn't white. This was Ireland in the '50s where the idea of a fine upstanding Catholic girl consorting with someone of color was frowned upon. Also assumed, and probably true, "black" students, being more affluent, offered women a more upscale experience than most of their white counterparts.

Other venues infrequently visited were the Crystal, off Grafton Street and Metropole on O'Connell Street. This, the largest and most popular of Dublin's dance halls, drew its clientele mainly from Dublin city and the north side of town. The downside, other than being pricey, was the significant walk back to the opposite side of the city after seeing someone home. And the peck on the cheek, often the only reward for your efforts, didn't shorten the distance. Bus service was not available after midnight.

More refined dance venues were found at the tennis clubs in the Ballsbridge and Rathmines sections of town. My recollection is of a clubby, family-connected cohort, whose social circle didn't extend beyond the Dublin Canal. Everyone was pleasant and the girls were pretty and well put out, but as charismatic and charming as I might have been, not being a member of their set placed me outside the pale. The superior quality of the music at these clubs - a live band, often five to six pieces, and a vocalist - easily trumped the amateurish offerings in other halls. An exception was the ensemble of Humphrey Murphy. Their size - a trio - and lack of sophistication was admirably off-set by repertoire, enthusiasm, and Humphrey's keyboard virtuosity.

The "Arts" was also popular for a more significant reason: most of the women who attended usually lived in the immediate area. Local or not, on learning that they lived at home, interest cooled, and an exit strategy was put in place. If, however, the woman had a flat or bed-sitter, there was potential. And if, by some stroke of good fortune she invited you in, you knew that your stars had finally aligned. There are memories of those nights, especially in spring and summer, when around four o'clock in the morning, all the birds in the area, with nary a warning chirp, erupted in a cacophony of song. From whatever couch, bed, or sofa you were stretched out upon, you knew it was time to head home.

At that point, varying degrees of hangover were evident. A by-product of this condition was often a terrible thirst. The only other activity occurring that time of morning were horse-drawn wagons making milk deliveries. The horses knew the routes so well that the driver, having tied the reins to the hansom, walked alongside the slowly-moving wagon and made his deliveries. With good timing, a pint or two of milk was easily off-loaded, the driver totally unaware of the heist. Even if seen, he only shouted after you. Milk, probably abetted by the thrill of the theft, never tasted so good. If a long distance had yet to be traveled, one was alert for an unattended bicycle. Inside a gate or leaned against the side of a garage, an unchained bike was considered fair game. With some stealth, you wheeled it outside the yard and off you went, the bicycle later left a discrete distance from the digs. These activities are mentioned, not to be condoned, but rather to illustrate the resourcefulness that was brought to bear in times of untoward circumstance.

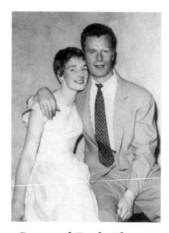

Gene and Freda Blaney
Arcadia Ballroom - Bray, 1956

Sometimes relationships lasted more than a few hours. If things seemed to be going well with a young lady and a certain ineffable chemistry was afoot, another meeting might be suggested. But one moved cautiously in these situations – the choice of words crucial, lest the wrong impression be given. The notion of a formal date, such as a movie or dinner, was never suggested or intimated. The thinking was more akin to a military operation: you wanted only to establish a beachhead and then consider your next assault. You weren't in a hurry to win the war. "It would be nice to get together sometime," would be an appropriate overture to the woman. To indicate the depth of your interest, you requested her phone number.

Money, or the lack thereof, was the limiting factor. Ten shillings would not cover drinks and a meal for two. When explaining your plight, if extremely understanding, the young lady might respond: "Why don't you drop by my flat next Friday, after the pubs close, if you've nothing planned?" This, the ideal situation, made for a relaxed Friday, as the pressure was off as to post-pub activities.

However, such was rarely the case. So, as closing approached, with phone numbers in hand, a telephone call or two was made. Whatever woman answered, you suggested that it might be fun to get together for a chat, as it had been awhile. If she thought so also, a couple of small whiskeys were pocketed and you headed off. Many of the women were from the country, and food sent by their parents often was available. After you chatted, enjoyed the whiskeys, and the well-stocked larder, attempts were made to enjoy the, hopefully, well-stacked owner of the larder. When taking your leave, you attempted, as discretely as possible, to ascertain when the next shipment of food was due, and as any prudent man would, you planned accordingly.

The Irish and their zealous consumption of alcohol have endured a long association. From the anecdotal accounts of English landlords, fearful for their safety when their Irish tenants "took to the drink," to "Paddy" wagons and the bulbous characterizations on stage and in film, a perception exists that somewhere in the Celtic DNA a fragment lurks which accounts for this affinity.

As a student in Dublin during the late 1950s and early 1960s, this history and its genetic implications were of little concern. The pub, for many of us, served a more immediate utility: an arena for social activity. Here we congregated and established friendships, which, often late in the evening, were vowed to be lifelong. It was a place where exam success was celebrated and failures softened, where stratagems for crashing parties were hatched, where songs were sung, and on Friday and Saturday nights, where camaraderie and conviviality reigned. Each of the major colleges had their local: Hartigan's on Leeson's Street for UCD, the Lincoln Inn just outside Trinity's back gate, and the Toby Jug for the College of Surgeons.

During those years, the hours of pub operations were limited. Most opened for business at noon, and except for an hour in the afternoon, remained so until 10:00 p.m. during the winter months and 10:30 p.m. through the summer. The afternoon closing - "the holy hour" - gave the owner a chance to clear the premises and prepare for the evening trade. A publican who served drinks to the public during this time was subject to a fine. This regulation was regularly circumvented in countless pubs across the city, where patrons, huddled around their pints, sat in semi-darkness. Close attention was paid to the sounds of the street, alert to the Garda making their rounds, listening for the telltale tap of their baton as they approached. After a push on the locked door or a turn of the knob, their steps receded. Grins all around, pints were raised at having pulled a fast one on the authority. Still, the tavern keeper, ever wary, gestured for silence in case the officer got "cute" and doubled back.

A pub's closure at 10:00 or 10:30 p.m. was considered by many to be, not only premature, but an affront to a civilized populace - a Church-concocted penance. If, however, a pleasant drinking rhythm had been established, when it would be "a shame altogether" to lose a glow so carefully nurtured, Irish law was accommodating: you became a bona-fide traveler.

A licensing act established in the late 1800s permitted those who had traveled in "good faith" at least three miles from the place where they had spent the previous night, to be served food and drink beyond the customary hours. Establishments located in the foothills of the Wicklow mountains, south of Dublin, easily reached by car, had obtained licenses to serve this itinerant population. On arrival you were directed to a sign-in book which listed the names of the travelers, the origin of their journey and their eventual destination, formally establishing credibility in case of inspection by the police. Eamon DeValera, Kevin Barry, Brian Boru, and Oliver Cromwell were some of the more prominent and frequently noted travelers. "Grangegorman," (a mental hospital), "to hell and Connemara," "a little piece down the road," and "beyond the pale" were popular destinations. The proprietor left remnants of meals strategically placed around the premises to create the illusion of food consumption.

Weekend crowds often exceeded the pub's capacity, especially if a sporting event was on in Dublin. The gathering congealed in a wedge of bodies around the bar, shrouded in smoke; conversations, absorbed in the drone, were reduced to shouts. Causalities of the night were evident: a young man propped in a chair in a corner of the room, head tilted against his chest, body unmoving, or another: white shirt stained with stout, face devoid of color, sprawled on a square of grass outside the establishment. No one paid them the slightest heed.

The bona fides remained open as long as travelers required service. Usually the last call was around 1:00 a.m., with the establishment vacated by 2:00 a.m. A parade of vehicles gathered for the trek to Dublin, a journey perilous enough to induce sobriety. Down twisted mountain roads the cavalcade careened through towns and villages, past pinpoints of light from tucked-in homes, to the orange-illuminated highway that led to the city.

For most, the arrival in Dublin signaled the end of the evening's activities. Others, not quite ready to quit the night, headed to what were called "speakeasies" during America's Prohibition Era - places where alcohol was served illegally.

One of the better known (where women of the night were said to work), was Dolly Fawcett's, located on Dublin's north side, near the Rotunda, the national maternity hospital. Its entrance, unlighted, led to a small grocery store, its counters dimly outlined. In front of a display case, a trapdoor opened to stairs which led to the cellar. The "lounge" was a low-ceilinged, unadorned gritty space with unshaded lights attached to support beams. Two small cubbies, formally coal bins, each had a small table and chairs. Covered with a stained table cloth, a large round table filled the central space; two smaller tables were set against the wall opposite the cubbies. Altogether, it was a dismal, dank place which reeked of mold and old porter. The whiskey, the first sips of which caused an immediate shudder, was served in heavy white mugs or teacups by an old crone with a stained apron, tangled hair and the occasional missing tooth.

As the night progressed, a younger version, similarly garbed and equally disheveled appeared and joined one of the tables where the men chatted her up and bestowed attention as if she were Maude Gonne herself (a legendary beauty and the unrequited love of W.B. Yeats). Scant attention was paid to our group, probably because of our youth and not being regular attendees of the establishment.

The night sky was lightening as we exited Dolly's. After the long night, food became an imperative; at that hour it was only available at the cattle markets located at the edge of town, near Kingsbridge railway station. Certain pubs were allowed to open at 4:00 a.m., accommodating farmers who had driven their cattle through the night for sale at the morning markets. For these legitimate travelers, breakfast and beverages were available. Entire families often accompanied the driver, or traveling by auto, joined in the morning. In contrast to our previous venue, we found ourselves in a large, bright, airy room, an expansion of the pub proper, where about twelve tables were set up for dining, half of which were occupied by the families. Haggard, unkempt and feeling totally out of place, we found a table at the back of the room.

The farmers were still involved with their livestock, so it was playtime for their fresh-faced children. Running between tables they had a grand time playing their version of hide and seek while their kerchiefed mothers chatted. Each mother dispensed snacks from a large wicker basket to hold over the hungry children until breakfast. Then the men arrived, garbed in heavy jackets or thick leather vests. Accompanying them were ruddy-faced young men with knee-high rubber boots caked with mud, who we presumed were their sons. With the children gathered, the families began their meal, prefaced with Grace. An occasional glance was given to the reprobates seated at the back of the room. The only remaining business for the cattle owner was the auction held later in the morning; the long night of his working day was over. Stout was available and flowed freely. For the ravenous all-night drinker, no breakfast could rival the eggs, ham, rasher, and sausage, eased down with a pint of stout, served at the cattle market pubs.

With bellies full, we made our way home, conversation muted by an overwhelming weariness. Finally: the digs, a crash into bed, and the end of a decent day's drinking in Dublin.

BRENDAN BEHAN

requently seen in Dublin during the late 1950s was the playwright, poet, author, and roustabout, Brendan Behan. A native of Dublin and a painter by trade, Brendan had achieved success with his plays, *Borstal Boy* and *The Hostage*. The former was written while incarcerated in England for activities as a member of the I.R.A. After his release he became associated with Joan Littlewood, the innovative director of a theater workshop in London, who produced plays, often avant-garde and controversial. Recognizing Brendan's "diamond in the rough" potential, she helped rework his abrasive syntax into a coherent vehicle for the stage. Acclaim followed, and Brendan, lifted from obscurity, became famous. His outsized persona was fueled by inordinate amounts of alcohol.

McDaid's, a pub off Grafton St., was Brendan's favorite, but not one to discriminate, he found comfort in a number of watering holes. Pat O'Brien and I were having a drink in Davy Byrnes one evening while Brendan was holding forth at the bar. For reasons we assumed to be inebriation, he toppled to the floor. An individual sitting opposite, well-dressed and proper in appearance, went over and began kicking Brendan, until pulled away. The man, a doctor as it turned out, offered no explanation other than he was sick of Brendan's obnoxious behavior.

Brendan was a diabetic and the diagnosis, it was said, had been made by a medical student drinking with him one night. After Brendan returned to the table, having relieved himself, the student noticed white flecks had formed around the splashes of urine on his shoes, which the student opined might be sugar. The diagnosis of diabetes was subsequently made.

Brendan's lifestyle and pathology impeded longevity. Barely forty-one when he lifted his last, his was an extravagant talent, scarcely tapped, done in by success and the "sauce."

A Harsh Winter
(But a Splendid Spring)

Christmas of 1956 was again spent with Tom Conneen in his rooms at Trinity. Tom was taking the "half" exams in Anatomy and Physiology around the end of March, but even at this juncture, was immersed in study for ten to twelve hours each day. Conversations with him, other than those dealing with the subject material were non-existent. Periodically, a movie was allowed.

The Dublin winter that followed was a particularly unrelenting time of cold and dampness, maintained without respite through a depressingly harsh January and February. March teased with a day or two of wan sunlight and then withdrew; April, with light lingering longer, made tentative overtures. Finally May, and as though a switch had been turned, spring arrived. Swards of green replaced the brown cover of Stephens Green, emerald shoots, encouraged by a scarcely remembered warmth, emerged in the gardens: the benches again were occupied. Forgotten was the misery of the winter past.

Tom Conneen passed his "half" exams (as if there were doubt), and traveled home to Maine. Exam success secured my admission into the second year of medical school.

Aunt Bertha was pleased with my progress and also felt it impractical that I return home, the cost of the voyages being the main consideration. With the summer free, she felt I should take advantage of the opportunity to see as much of Europe as possible. Money was forwarded along with literature regarding youth hostels, Euro-rail information, and suggested places to visit. I thought it a great idea.

An In-flight Emergency

My flight to Europe originated in London. Munich was the destination, and the aircraft was a two-engine, propeller-driven relic, probably a DC6 or DC7. Midway through the flight, the captain announced that radio communications with the ground had been lost; a holding pattern would be maintained until the situation was resolved.

As an addendum: beverages, including wine and beer, were available, without cost, as an apology for the delay. As luck would have it, I was seated next to a fine looking, blonde woman, a fortunate diversion during this time of peril. My initial conversational foray was, I felt, quite glib.

"The only way to fly," I ventured. "Free drinks, a good-looking woman, and no one knows where we are."

Expecting a haughty look and a return to the book in her lap, I was surprised by her laugh and the smile that followed.

"Well, that does add a little drama to the trip, doesn't it?"

While the plane lazily circled broad banks of sun-splashed clouds, our conversation, mellowed by beer, flowed easily. Eva informed me, in excellent English, that she taught German at a secondary school in England.

"I'm headed home for the summer."

"Munich?" I asked.

"No, a small village about a hundred kilometers to the north."

"Anything exciting planned or just a lazy time off?"

"Well, yes, at least pretty exciting for me. I'm getting married in August."

"Congratulations, or I guess I should say good wishes to the female."

"I'll take either. Thank you."

She told me her fiancé lived in the same village and together they would return to England to live and work: he, as an engineer, having just completed his degree.

Ground-to-air communications were restored, and the plane landed late that afternoon, almost two hours behind schedule. As a result, Eva missed her train connection home. Familiar with the city, she knew of reasonably priced hotels.

We shared a taxi into Munich, a city I knew little about other than it having been one of the more heavily bombed targets during WW II. This also was the city where Hitler achieved his first significant notoriety; his ill-fated beer-hall putsch. Entering the inner city everything seemed new, and indeed it was, with most of the bombed buildings razed and replaced with modern structures. In the old section of town, however, blocks of destruction still remained with demolition and reconstruction on-going.

After Eva chatted with the driver regarding hotel locations, she turned to me. "You know," she said, "I think it's foolish to pay for two rooms when we could share one and split the bill. What do you think?"

Not wishing to stammer, I spoke slowly. "I think it is a splendid idea, a really splendid idea." So share a room we did.

That night, after Eva telephoned home, we enjoyed a meal and a few more beers. On our return to the room my overtures were accepted, until I began an exploration of previously admired territory.

She pulled away. "It's something of an awkward moment for me right now."

"Awkward?" Even accented, her English was very proper.

"Not a good time." She paused. "And I really don't want to make a mess. Also," she added quickly, "I'm engaged and I don't feel I should ..."

I interrupted. "Say no more. I'm not in the mood anyway."

She laughed. "Now I know *that's* a lie."

So, we chatted on a multitude of topics, shared some bad jokes and enjoyed each other until overtaken by sleep. In the morning we showered and breakfasted on croissants and coffee. Her blonde hair, still moist and twisted into a clip at the top of her head, gave off the perfume of shower gel.

During the cab ride to the train station, we recounted the serendipity of our meeting; an encounter, we agreed, that would hardly be remembered, but perhaps not totally forgotten - an unexpected vignette to tease the memory. At the station - a hug, then she entrained north and I south.

From Munich, with my railway pass, I traveled through the Garmisch area of southern Germany, truly beautiful country, even if only appreciated through the window of a moving train. A train change was required in Linz, then on to Innsbruck, Austria where I stayed the night. The following morning, in tourist fashion, I checked out the town and later boarded a train that ascended the fabled Brenner Pass into Italy and on to Rome.

After an overnight in Rome, I boarded a train to Venice the following morning. The scene on the train was predictably chaotic: crowded, with babies crying, suitcases strewn about, food consumed from large baskets, the smell of fruit. Falling asleep, I awoke to find I had missed the Venice stop and was half-way to Trieste, Yugoslavia. Trieste, at that time, was Communist-controlled. On my arrival, the authorities examined my passport, gave me twenty four hours to vacate the city, which I did with haste, leaving on the next available train back to Venice.

Once there, I located a room in the Lido section of the city, near the beaches. Lacking a bathing suit, I found a relatively uninhabited section of the strand, where a swim, in all my naked glory, was enjoyed in water much warmer than at home.

The following morning I made my way around Venice and found it to be a unique city. Built on a series of interconnected islands, transportation was accomplished primarily by gondola and power boats of varying sizes. Its dominance as a maritime port was established during the Crusades when necessities (food stuffs, ships and crew - required to continue the journey to the Holy Land), were provided by Venetian merchants. As a consequence, Venice became, at that time, the richest city in the world. I was struck that morning by the magnificent homes which lined the canals, perched so precariously; water lapped at the door-steps, their continued existence completely dependent on the vagaries of the Mediterranean tide.

Attaching myself to a guided tour, I saw much of the city: Marco Polo's birthplace; the red light district along the appropriately named "Via de Teat"; the Bridge of Sighs, so named because it lead to the prison; the Piazza San Marco, fronting the spectacular multi-domed Basilica; and the Clock Tower, presenting a panoramic view of the city, its chimes scattering pigeons on the plaza below. In true tourist fashion I had a Bellini - champagne and peach juice - at "Harry's Bar." This was a hang-out for the glitterati of the social and screen set, made famous (and its future secured), by Ernest Hemingway's frequent attendance and the mentions of the bar in his novels.

The morning of the third day I made my return to Rome.

By chance, the youth hostel where I stayed was located two blocks from the Coliseum which I explored the next morning. With the movie *Roman Holiday* as my guide, I attempted to locate some of the places Gregory Peck, darting about the city on his Vespa, had brought Audrey Hepburn. I did find the wall to which hundreds of petitions to the Blessed Mother were affixed but otherwise met with little success. Following narrow cobbled streets in rather haphazard fashion, I came upon the arch of Titus, Trajan's Column, and the Pantheon. There I attached myself to a tour group and learned that the marble used in its construction was from Egypt, and the coffered concrete dome formed a perfect sphere – diameter equal to height. During the hunt for the Catacombs I became hopelessly lost.

An interesting recollection relates to the Roman method of bladder relief. Men, either walking along the sidewalk or having hopped off their bikes, went to a portion of a wall along the sidewalk, identified only by a plaque titled "Pissoir." There they did their thing and went their way. The small sign and the trough which led to the street were the only indications of its function.

Around noon I stopped for lunch at a small restaurant, off the beaten tourist path. Three of the half-dozen tables were occupied, one by a young female wearing glasses, reading a book, with a beverage at her side. I sat at the table next to her. The waiter brought a menu. As I hoped, my indecision regarding food selection was noted by the woman.

"Language problem?" she asked. Her accent was definitely American.

I nodded. "The only things I recognize are pizza and spaghetti bolognaise."

She laughed. "I know the feeling."

When she turned, I could see her book's title: *Moral Theology*.

"Pretty heavy reading you're doing there," I said.

"Yes," she nodded. "Hard slogging."

"I went through my share of it. Had the Jesuits for four years and that stuff's right in their wheel-house."

The conversation continued as I enjoyed my pizza. Terry, short for Teresa, spoke about her experience with nuns in high school and her impressions of Rome after a month in the city. I recollected my days at Holy Cross and something of my medical school experience in Ireland. Chatting provided the opportunity to check out the physical package: blonde hair cut short, without apparent concern for fashion, and a pale complexion (lacking make-up). Her sparkling blue eyes and ready smile were an attractive counterpoint to an otherwise serious mien. Although probably influenced by my morning outing, she had the fragile look of Mr. Peck's Audrey. The areas of my libidinal curiosity were obscured, however, by a wide white cotton skirt that fell to her ankles and a loose teal-green blouse that disguised any prominences.

"Have you seen much of Rome?" she wondered.

"Hardly scratched the surface, but I really want to get to St. Peter's – for reasons more architectural than spiritual."

"Then I'll take you there. I know it well."

"You've been there; you'll be bored to tears."

"Maybe, but it beats moral theology," she laughed. "I'm a great guide; you'll learn all kinds of interesting things. Let's go."

And off we went. Terry was correct. Before the sun set over Rome that night, I was party to a startling revelation, in fact, a divinely inspired one...

As we walked across the wide, column-encircled piazza toward the basilica of St. Peter, Terry pointed out the balcony where the Pope makes his appearances and the chimney of the

Sistine Chapel from which trails of white smoke announce the selection of a new Pope.

Wide doors at the rear of the portico opened to a vast nave lined with altars on each side. At the far end was a raised altar below a draped canopy.

"Beneath this polished floor is where St. Peter is buried," she said. "Don't know how they know for sure," she added, "as it was a graveyard back then with many bodies. Divine inspiration, maybe," she said, smiling.

Multiple groups of tourists were being escorted by guides and although my usual strategy was to hook onto one, Terry easily assumed the role. She discussed in some detail the background of many of the statues, altars, and artifacts. (I've forgotten most of the details, but I do remember Michelangelo's Pieta – Mary holding the dead Jesus in her arms – and the statue of St. Peter, the toes of his right foot worn down by centuries of tourists who traditionally touch the foot as they pass.)

We took a slow, creaky elevator to the base of the free-standing dome, totally supported by its own weight, and from there climbed a narrow wooden spiral staircase to its top. Far below was the broad piazza with its central obelisk and on every side, Rome spread out before us – a magnificent panorama. Later when I mentioned to Terry my intention to see the Sistine Chapel, she asked if I would mind visiting it alone.

"I've seen it many times, Gene," she said. "I just want to sit for awhile."

The chapel was crowded and noisy, and though I did admire Michelangelo's work, it was more for reasons of reputation than art appreciation. At that time many of the ceiling scenes were smudged, discolored, and obscured by the ravages of time. (It wasn't until years later when a major renovation of the ceiling had been accomplished that the color and detail were restored to the masterpiece.)

I returned to meet Terry. She wasn't where I had left her.

Then I saw her kerchiefed profile, kneeling at one of the side altars, hands clasped; her face, alabaster in the gray light was fixed on the cross before her. After a few minutes I went over and tapped her on the shoulder. Looking up, she stared at me intently for a few seconds, as though waking from sleep, then stood up and we left.

The decision was unanimous, after the long afternoon and the heat that is Rome in the summer, it was time to hoist a cool beer. We found a small café, out of the sun, across the street from the Trevi fountain.

I lifted my drink toward her. "Cincin. Thanks for the tour. It was a great afternoon."

Our glasses touched.

"I enjoyed it, too," she said.

Across the square, groups of people were in constant flux. We had great fun guessing the nationalities of the tourists by their garb and behavior, and our accompanying comments, though not charitable, we agreed were dead-on. Terry had a great sense of humor.

Another round was ordered. After my lame, "Here's looking at you, Kid," I asked, "Why don't you join me for supper. After all you've done, it's the least I can do. And maybe you could introduce me to something other than spaghetti bolognaise. How about it?"

She looked at me for a moment. "No, I don't think so, Gene." She took a draught of beer and added, "There's something you should know about me."

"What's that?"

"I'm a nun."

"You're joking, right?"

"No, I'm not."

I was stunned. I knew there was something different about her, but never suspected this – though I guess the clues had been there.

"I would have told you earlier, but I didn't want to spend the rest of the afternoon answering questions. Plus, I enjoyed being an anonymous young woman with a young man again."

"It's all fine, Terry, just wasn't expecting it. Taken aback as they say in England."

"I'm sure you are."

She took a sip of her drink, then clasping her hands together, leaned over the table.

"Let me tell you something of my story. I'll be brief."

I nodded.

"About two years after high school graduation, I entered the Sisters of Mercy novitiate in Michigan, not too far from where I grew up. I'll spare you the details that led to the decision. When I said a moment ago that I was a nun, it wasn't totally true. Last spring I finished my third year in the novitiate and professed my first vows. In another three years, with the help of God, I'll profess my second, and three years later, the final perpetual commitment. Those who have reached this first step are invited to Rome for two months to study, pray, and share the contemplative life of the sisters living in the diocese here. The novitiate provides room, board, and a small stipend. My family came up with the airfare. So here I am."

"Incredible," I said. "Are you happy? What will you do when you finish?"

"Yes, I'm very happy. I'll either teach or work with the poor."

"But you're a nun. What are you doing having a beer with a man you barely know?"

"I like men, always have, but I must say it's been awhile since I've had a beer with one."

"I'm honored, Sister." The sarcasm produced a smile. "Did you ever think about leaving – quitting?"

"Used to...frequently. In fact, I left once for a while and hooked up with an old boyfriend. Back to the old days - poverty, chastity and obedience took a holiday. But no matter how hard

I partied, no matter how much I drank, it kept calling me back."

"What did?"

"God's love. There's no escaping, you know. No matter where you hole up, it'll find you. Then one day I couldn't take it anymore. It was surrender time. And I did. I went back." She paused. "And I'll never leave again."

"Reminds me of the old negro spiritual," I said. "No use a'runnin', when the Lord's a'comin'.'"

"I never heard that. But did you ever read *The Hound of Heaven*? 'I fled him down the days and down the nights...down the labyrinthine ways of my mind...'"

"Don't think so," I replied.

"You should – Francis Thompson – his poem explains it far better than I'm able." She looked at her watch. "Must be going, Gene, we have evening prayers in about an hour." She stood up to leave.

"Not much point in saying we'll keep in touch, is there, Terry?"

"No, we'll never see each other again. But we'll always have a nice day to remember. And good luck to you back in Ireland."

We hugged, then standing on her tip-toes, she placed a wisp of a kiss on my cheek, then turned away. As she began to merge into the sidewalk traffic I thought she might look back and give a wave. She didn't.

I sat down and ordered another beer. "I swear," I thought to myself, "I've no luck at all."

The following morning I checked out of the hostel, bused to the train station, and using my Euro-pass, booked passage on the mid-afternoon express to Monaco. I had acquired a painful tooth, an increasing distraction, the discomfort only partially relieved by Veganin, an over-the-counter aspirin-strength pain reliever.

Located in the principality of Monaco, the casino at Monte Carlo, a multi-columned, stone structure, library-like in appearance, was impressive. Inside, tuxedoed croupiers presided over the tables. Seated behind stacks of colored chips, players made their wagers - drinks and cigarette by their side. Although early evening, most were well-turned out: ladies in cocktail dresses, gentlemen in suits. The scene, accompanied by the variety of accents, lent an air of intrigue. Around 7:00 p.m. I was approached by a man wearing a badge and asked to leave. The reason: my lack of proper attire.

Dismissed but hardly fazed, I reasserted my sophistication at the adjacent Hotel de Paris, where I sipped an extraordinarily expensive beer at a multi-mirrored, leather-bound bar, lined with beautiful people. When I placed my order, the formally-attired bartender appraised rather than welcomed me; his thin lips poised between smile and derision as he considered whether I was worthy of his services. When I finished my drink, in a small gesture of defiance, I raised my glass and with a subtle inclination of my torso, wished him a good evening.

Nice, six miles east and also on the coast, was disappointing - at least the beaches were. The shoreline, ringed by hotels, and the surrounding hills studded with beautiful homes, offered an extravagant backdrop to a blue, sun-bathed Mediterranean, dotted with sailboats and motor craft. Along the shore, however, long stretches of rock-strewn terrain extended to the water's edge. Beach-goers who wished to lie or sit on the shore, of necessity, employed inflatable cushions and mattresses. The comparison to the long, sandy beaches in New England was obvious.

My dental discomfort persisted to the point where I needed to find relief. Directed by a pharmacist, I located a dentist who would see me at the end of her appointments that day. Certain she could help until I returned to Ireland, she anesthetized the area, drilled out the decay and placed a temporary filling. The procedure took about ten minutes. The dentist, an older lady, probably in her sixties, spoke English well. When I requested a bill for her services she demurred, citing the minor procedure. After some conversation, I asked if she would at least join me for a glass of wine. Declining, she explained that friends were arriving for supper but suggested I come along, as one of the couples was headed to the United States in the next day or two.

I hesitated. I'd planned on taking the late train to Paris and didn't want to miss it. After explaining my indecision, the dentist insisted I'd be at the station in plenty of time. So I gratefully accepted her invitation. For reasons that became apparent later, it was a most fortuitous decision.

The discussion, over a delicious supper of fresh tomatoes, cheese, and avocado salad, revolved around the United States and the upcoming trip. The couple, a husband and wife, were making their first transatlantic plane journey, with San Francisco their final destination. When, during the course of the conversation, I mentioned I was headed to Paris, the husband, after a moment of conversation with his wife, turned to me.

"Excuse my English," he began, "our car we sold to a dealer nearby Paris and it is..." He paused. "Comment dites-vous en Anglais? An advantage," he continued, "if vous..." He shook his head and talked directly with the dentist for a minute or so in French.

After their conversation, Anna, I believe was her name, told me the couple had sold their car to a dealership outside Paris. "They wonder if you would consider driving the car to the dealer. It would save them considerable expense - not having to hire a driver and transport him back. What do you think?"

"I'd be glad to do it," I replied, "except I don't have an international driver's license."

Anna spoke again with the husband, then turned to me. "Apparently a license from any state in your country is acceptable."

"In that case, they've got a driver."

In the morning, arrangements were made, and provided with petrol money, the Renault and I started our journey of about 500 miles. From Nice the route took us through Provence (a flat countryside, interrupted by vast vineyards), to Lyon for a lunch break, and after crossing the fabled Rhone River, so began the long haul to Paris. Progress was interrupted by a sudden cloud burst at which time I discovered the wind-shield wiper on the driver's side to be inoperative. Fortunately, I found refuge beneath an overpass until the rains passed - one white wall of which proclaimed the extraordinary sexual talents of a certain "Celeste." I arrived late in the evening, only to discover that the dealership was closed. I arranged lodging for the night and delivered the car in the morning.

The manager asked, in broken English, "Do you have any problems? Car run good?" He didn't ask how I happened to be driving it.

"Great car," I replied, "no problems." I didn't consider the wind-shield wiper worthy of mention. After accepting a ride to the station, a commuter train deposited me in Paris. My intention was to visit my friends in Val d'Or, but I decided instead to head directly to Dublin.

What made the episode noteworthy, related to the famous Blue Train that commuted regularly between Nice and Paris, and which I had planned to take that evening. Sometime during the night a portion of the train went off the track injuring many; two or three passengers were killed. My dental miseries were well-timed and may have prevented an untoward event.

The trip was a nice break in the action. Bertha provided the bulk of the money for the excursion but my mother also contributed. Whenever I wrote to her, the return letter always, without fail, contained money. They both believed, even my mother who never went anywhere, that when you traveled, you learned, and what you learned could be just as important as a school experience. For their generosity, I was grateful.

The Second Medical Year

We began our second medical year with approximately twelve less classmates. The curriculum, a continuation of the first year's Anatomy and Physiology, would be completed in approximately six months, at which time the "half" exam was taken. If passed, entry into the clinical years commenced.

As the year progressed, my routine remained unchanged. Life in the digs kept to its usual pattern, the core group fixed, with only the occasional interloper. My consistently unexciting social life persisted. Study habits were maintained, albeit somewhat erratically, until about four weeks prior to an exam. At that point things academic ratcheted up. More attention was paid in class, better notes were taken, while attendance at the UCD library became more punctual and regular. The National Library on Kildare Street, to which I had been recently introduced, became a frequent destination.

There was a cadre of students whose approach to exams - because of the chutzpa and derring-do involved - set them apart from the mainstream sloggers. Their premise hinged on the concept of intellectual frugality: only expend enough effort in exam preparation to ensure a passing grade - be only as smart as you had to be. More extravagant efforts were reserved only for those situations when truly under the gun. In their view, if one were asked how an exam turned out and one responded, "Yeh, got it, just slipped by," and pulled it off consistently - that was much more impressive than achieving Honors. Though their model of scholastic endeavor was not one I aspired to, it was, nevertheless, my inclination.

The exam format at Surgeons, similar to other institutions at that time, was, in my opinion, something of a crap shoot as far as determining one's knowledge of a subject. It was geared more to failure than success: written exams consisting of eight to twelve essay-type questions. Considering the scope of the subjects (anatomy and physiology, for instance), passing, determined by these few questions, spoke more to good fortune than an understanding of the material. A multiple-choice test format, covering a wider spectrum, would have been a better indicator of knowledge, and could have removed luck from the equation. I'm sure that's the method in place currently. And probably if I were a student today, I'd want the old format back.

Christmas that year was a dour affair. Tom Conneen spent the holiday with his roommate in England; Miss Halligan visited her family for the week, closing the digs. At that time I was seeing Doreen, a young lady whom I met at a dance, who early one morning introduced me to "The Ballad of Reading Gaol" ("... for each man kills the thing he loves, by all let this be heard...") and the genius of Oscar Wilde. Leaving for the holidays, Doreen generously let me use her apartment on Earlsfort Terrace, off Adelaide Road. Neighbors included Micheál mac Liammóir, the celebrated Irish actor in *The Importance of Being Oscar*, playing at the time, and his partner, Hilton Edwards.

The elephants in the room, as the holidays wound down, were the upcoming exams in Anatomy and Physiology. I resolved that the New Year would inaugurate a more focused study routine.

After eighteen months, the dreaded Anatomy and Physiology exams were upon us. Legions of careers had floundered attempting to overcome these twin monsters – the Scylla and Charybdis of the curriculum – who patrolled the entrance to the world of clinical medicine. Once safely through their clutches, the odds of completing the second half of the syllabus, if not guaranteed, could be reasonably assumed. As alluded to earlier, the mountains of material culled to a dozen questions for each subject, would delight the heart of any bookmaker. Passing on the initial effort restored one's faith more in the power of prayer, than the efficacy of diligent study. To preen and admit to a superior acumen, if thus favored, was flirting with delusion. One could also look forward to a relatively relaxed spring and summer with first-try success.

My exam preparation was in turn, intense and sporadic – directly related to the level of anxiety that was aboard at any given time. I enjoyed physiology compared to its "anatomical" mate. The logic, the complexity, the inter-play between systems appealed to me. It just seemed to make sense. (Years later I met an academic physician who told me that he was an atheist until he began post-graduate studies in physiology. Delving into the elaborate mechanisms that maintain our existence convinced him of the presence of an intelligent design, a force – name optional – that created our planet and the cosmos beyond. Pulverizing a Swiss watch and injecting the specks of material into a vast universe, then expecting the fragments, on their own, to recreate a complex timepiece, was in his phrase, "Bullshit." His analogy, specious as it might be, made sense to me.)

Between the written exams and orals in both subjects, along with a viva in Anatomy and a lab in Physiology, it was a four day event. The night before the written exam, a fellow student produced a list of what she guaranteed to be the questions on the Anatomy paper. She said "a friend" was the source of the acquisition. Four or five of us spent hours that night feverishly going over the questions. A portion of one question, I remember, concerned the origin, course, and structures innervated by the phrenic nerve. Naturally, not one of the questions appeared on the exam. A good night's sleep would have been of greater benefit.

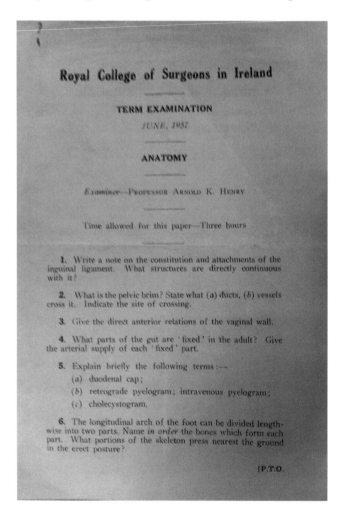

Royal College of Surgeons in Ireland

TERM EXAMINATION

JUNE, 1957

ANATOMY

Examiner—Professor Arnold K. Henry

Time allowed for this paper—Three hours

1. Write a note on the constitution and attachments of the inguinal ligament. What structures are directly continuous with it?

2. What is the pelvic brim? State what (a) ducts, (b) vessels cross it. Indicate the site of crossing.

3. Give the direct anterior relations of the vaginal wall.

4. What parts of the gut are 'fixed' in the adult? Give the arterial supply of each 'fixed' part.

5. Explain briefly the following terms :—
   (a) duodenal cap;
   (b) retrograde pyelogram; intravenous pyelogram;
   (c) cholecystogram.

6. The longitudinal arch of the foot can be divided lengthwise into two parts. Name in order the bones which form each part. What portions of the skeleton press nearest the ground in the erect posture?

[P.T.O.

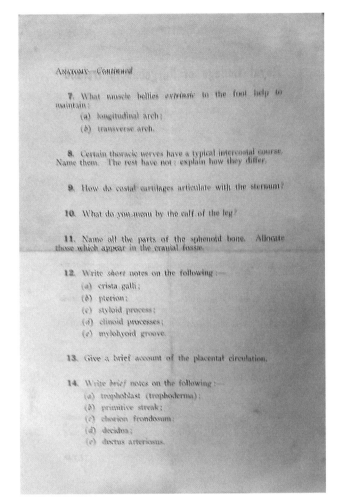

ANATOMY—Continued

7. What muscle bellies *extrinsic* to the foot help to maintain:
    (a) longitudinal arch;
    (b) transverse arch.

8. Certain thoracic nerves have a typical intercostal course. Name them. The rest have not: explain how they differ.

9. How do costal cartilages articulate with the sternum?

10. What do you mean by the calf of the leg?

11. Name all the parts of the sphenoid bone. Allocate those which appear in the cranial fossae.

12. Write *short* notes on the following :—
    (a) crista galli;
    (b) pterion;
    (c) styloid process;
    (d) clinoid processes;
    (e) mylohyoid groove.

13. Give a brief account of the placental circulation.

14. Write *brief* notes on the following :—
    (a) trophoblast (trophoderma);
    (b) primitive streak;
    (c) chorion frondosum;
    (d) decidua;
    (e) ductus arteriosus.

Sample of Exam Format

The actual exams seemed anti-climactic, almost a relief after all the studying, comparable to a marathon after months of training. Avoiding major gaffes, I felt reasonably confident at the finish. Two days later the official notification: I had passed.

Jettisoning these two exams in March afforded a significant window before the new medical year commenced in October. Introductory Pathology, Psychology and Practical Pharmacology lectures were scheduled during that period, none of which would include an exam. Although not yet decided, going home for the summer seemed a pretty good bet. Also, my participation in sports had been pretty much non-existent. This would be a good chance to get involved in some activity. The rowing club was recruiting, and although I had no experience it sounded like fun. I'd at least look into it.

But first: success in any exam required a celebratory response, certainly a mandate considering the significance of those just completed. An appropriate amount of cash was required to ensure a decent night. To this end, I hauled my anatomy and physiology texts to their new home - a local pawn shop. The few pounds I received softened the loss of my erstwhile, dog-eared bookmates.

(Similar transactions were conducted through my remaining years at Surgeons. The only books in my possession today which indicate my presence in Ireland are Bailey and Lowe's Surgery and a Conybeare & Mann medical text, the latter worn beyond resale value.)

As a student in Dublin during the 1960s, I developed an expedient association with this venerable institution. Just as it does now, the pawnshop functioned as a cash exchange for various commodities, either sold directly to the shop or left to be redeemed at a later date. The transactions were accomplished with a modicum of time and technicality.

Raised in a middle-class family, I had scant knowledge of this commerce but nonetheless had acquired the assumption that the pawn shop was the final refuge of the truly downtrodden and the place where gangsters fenced their ill-gotten goods. As a youngster I remember peering in the windows of our town's only pawn shop, seeing watches and jewelry displayed on a colored cloth backdrop, with musical instruments, cradled in velvet cases, propped in the corner. My adolescent imagination pictured gifted jazzmen bartering the tools of their craft for drugs; or desperate women, beautiful and bereft of inhibition, selling jewels for just one more roll of the dice.

These melodramas were less ominous during times of financial necessity. In fact, a sense of security pervaded, when my Holy Cross ring garnered three pounds and ten shillings, and a Tissot watch, a college graduation present from my grandmother, fetched four pounds. When my financial ship came in, they were reclaimed, for an additional ten shillings.

One day after an unsuccessful negotiation at an inner city pawn shop, I was directed to an establishment on Richmond Street, a working-class neighborhood. The building presented a plain facade without the trademark balls hanging above the entrance. The business area, a large room with a counter extending its length, was partitioned at one end into three cubicles for private negotiation. Behind the counter stood the owner, Paddy, a tall man, face creased and gaunt, probably in his sixties. A felt hat sat high on his forehead; suspenders, drawn down over a white shirt, were fixed to his trousers. A cigarette dangled from his mouth, his head tilted to let the smoke snake by. Two young boys worked with him, storing the pawned merchandise and making the occasional transaction.

The role of the pawn shop as an economic necessity was most apparent on Monday mornings. Then the shop was filled to overflowing, sometimes onto the sidewalk, as women pawned the family's dress-up Sunday clothes, until reclaimed with Friday's paycheck.

Some women arrived with clothes draped over their arms, shoes tied together and slung over their shoulders; others pushed prams, filled with garments. Jockeying for position they awaited negotiations with Paddy. The scene was bedlam. Young children ran loose; babies cried. Occasional strings of curses pierced the constant cackle of conversation. Standing tall above the fray and in total control was Paddy. As a priest in the confessional, he listened to tales of woe, heard countless times before, and after consideration, dispensed his indulgences. Paddy knew the regulars by name. And also the thread of their lives: Baptisms, First Communions, Confirmations, funerals, weddings - followed and remembered - by the clothes they brought to his shop.

This backdrop, coupled with the honed skills of the supplicants who cajoled and bargained in their tough Dublin accents, lent a theater atmosphere to a typical transaction.

"Ah Jasus, Paddy, don't you look grand today?" a woman chortled as she layered the counter with clothes, topped with a man's suit. A pair of shoes was placed off to the side.

"Good morning, Mary," said Paddy quietly. He quickly browsed the heap of clothes, checked the lining of the suit for tears, the shoe soles for holes.

"Fifteen shillings for the suit, ten for the shoes," Paddy intoned. "The rest I don't want."

"Ah, Paddy. Don't be teasing now; just be fair is all I'm feckin' askin. D'ya not see the fine press holding in the suit?"

"I've been seeing it for awhile, Mary. Hasn't changed." Paddy took a drag of his cigarette. "Don't waste my time this morning; I'm not in the mood."

"It's not for me, Paddy, but the baby. A little extra for the tot is all I'm askin."

"Now was it the tot you were thinking about when you bought your Woodbines, dear?" Paddy asked, nodding toward the cigarettes in her pocketbook. His pencil was poised over the claim tickets. "So what's it to be?"

"Jasus, you're a hard one." The woman leaned over the counter, her voice lowered. "Listen, Paddy, the old man's sick, ain't working, desperate he is."

"And would it be a recent illness, Mary?"

"Into a fortnight I'd guess."

"Then it wasn't him I saw last week having a pint in Mooney's, I suppose?" Paddy, feigning exasperation, looked to the ceiling. "You're trying my patience, Mary," he said. "It's twenty-five bob or off you go." Mary nodded yes.

Paddy scribbled on two tags. One he attached to the shoes, which he tossed onto a pile behind him; the other he affixed to the suit, which one of his helpers hung on a rack. Twenty-five shillings was pushed across the counter.

"God bless you, Paddy." Mary stuffed the money in her bag and pushed her way back through the crowd.

"Next," snapped Paddy.

"How'd it go, Mary?" a voice asked.

"Feckin' hair up his arse, has old Paddy," she muttered. "How d'ya think it went with that old bollocks?"

Over the years I came to know a little of Paddy. A decent man, he gave a fair price and didn't begrudge the extra shillings to those he felt were truly in need. He lamented their circumstance, the treadmill of their poverty, especially pertaining to the children who were likely to maintain the cycle. When I talked to "old ones" in line, they told of his giving back clothes, especially in winter, to families who couldn't redeem them.

Paddy lived by himself in the back room of the shop and by his own account, spent his nights sipping Powers whiskey, smoking Afton cigarettes, and watching the telly. His wife had died some years before, and he seldom saw his two sons; one lived in Mexico, the other in the United States. Making a few pounds above the rent, he was waiting for the day when he could sell the business, buy a cottage in Greystones; get the chance to put his feet up and watch the sea change color. Greystones, he explained, was a seaside resort in County Wicklow where, as a young boy, his family took their summer holiday.

(Before I left Dublin, I stopped to see Paddy one last time, my only visit with nothing to hock. He said he was sorry about the Tissot...the grandmother and all. (Paddy had acquired the Tissot and the class ring when circumstances were especially dire.) "Just to let you know," he added, "I made ten quid."

I smiled. "Good for you."

He wished me luck and we shook hands.)

Fifteen years later as I made my way along Richmond Street, new construction had altered the old landmarks. As closely as I could reconstruct the area in my mind, what formerly was the pawn shop and the adjoining stores had become a multi-storied brick building. But the pub across the street, despite fresh paint and tacky chrome ornamentation, seemed familiar as the one where I had often started the celebration of my new-found wealth.

The young lad behind the bar hadn't a clue when I inquired about the former buildings across the street. He referred me to an older man having a drink in the cubby at the end of the bar.

"Sure, I remember the pawn shop," the man said, accepting

my offer of a fresh pint. "Burned down some ten years ago, destroyed most of the block with it."

"And the owner, Paddy?" I asked.

"Died in the blaze. Started with a cigarette, the fire people said. Yeah, poor old Paddy. The funeral was in St. Kevins. All the old ones were there and the families he knew over the years. Packed the church they did. Everyone liked old Paddy." He paused. "Did you know him?"

"Years ago. I liked him too."

The old gentleman thanked me for the pint - said he was glad to be of help.

I haven't needed the services of a pawn shop since Dublin, yet whenever I pass one it is with some affection that I recall the shop on Richmond Street that saved the day so many times. As for Paddy...I'm only sorry that he never made it to that cottage in Greystones, to put his feet up and watch the sea change color.

The Rowing Adventure

Rowing was a traditional sport in most European colleges and universities at that time; in the US, more of a niche sport at Ivy League colleges. This has changed dramatically. American crews, from various parts of the country, have challenged and occasionally dominated their European counterparts.

In Dublin, the Blues of Trinity College were the premier team, followed by UCD and the Garda (police). If one considered pure muscle mass and strength as criteria, the Garda had no challengers. Simply to be a member of that organization required a minimum height of 6 feet and most had a complementary bulk. Once they became rowing fit, they were a force to be reckoned with, no matter the competition.

Dave Watkins was Surgeon's club president. Endeavoring to maintain the club's ranks, he was constantly recruiting. He persuaded me, along with classmates Pat O'Brien, Tom Lomas, Mike Thomas, and Paddy Hurley, to give it a shot. To my knowledge, with the exception of Mike Thomas, none of the group had rowed before. To say that Mr. Watkins had become desperate in his search would be an understatement.

Surgeons shared space with UCD in their boathouse at Islandbridge on the upper Liffey. At our disposal were single sculls, two- and four-man boats and a racing eight. Our equipment wasn't the caliber of other teams, as we weren't, but considering the whole package we didn't do badly. Dave was able to pry some funds out of the college coffers for a new (used) eight which was a significant up-grade.

We only participated in three or four major competitions: Galway, Belfast on the river Lagan, and Dublin's Head of the River. No trophies came our way but we competed, and speaking with considerable bias, acquitted ourselves admirably.

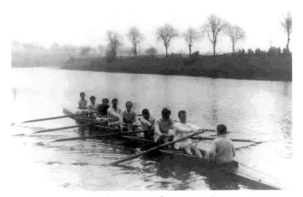

Positioning Boat for Race Start -
River Lagan, Belfast - 1959

Rowing was a demanding venture, certainly the most grueling team effort I've been involved with. Most crews were extremely fit, totally dedicated to the sport and the required training. Our group had a more flexible commitment. Race preparation involved occasional calisthenics, jogs through Phoenix Park, and rowing practices three times a week. Dave Watkins imposed a no smoking or drinking policy for some period prior to a race. Rather than risk a debilitating withdrawal, abstinence was down-graded to significant reduction. Mr. Watkins was not apprised of the modification.

The premier event was the annual Head of the River on Dublin's Liffey River. The race began at Islandbridge and finished at Butt Bridge in the center of Dublin, a distance of about three miles. The boat was carried over a weir to the starting point. Multiple crews were entered, with Trinity and UCD, the perennial local favorites.

Being one of the lighter crew members I rowed number eight, the stroke position. Tim Meagher, the coxswain, faced me. There were occasional changes in crew composition, but my recollection had Pat O'Brien in the number seven position, followed by Tom Lomas at number six. The power in the middle was supplied by Harri Lamki, Mike Thomas and a couple of burly underclassmen. Paddy Hurley occupied the number two position in the bow. Tim's job as cox was to keep us on course and advise regarding the stroke rate, dictated by our position in the race. My task was to establish the rate, maintain a consistent rhythm, and hopefully eight oars would strike the water at the same time.

The initial portion of the race was great fun. Spectators lined the wall overlooking the Liffey, shouting encouragement as the boats passed. But the fun quickly became an ordeal. Our crew was always trying to catch up; as a result, the stroke rate was frequently increased. Tim and I had the occasional strategy discussion.

"Gene, got to pick it up. Getting behind."

"You shitin' me? We're feckin' dying…"

"Just a bit. Almost there."

"Shut up."

The pace was picked up a notch.

Finally, legs cramped, arms burning, chests heaving, it was over. Slumped across our oars we drifted for a few minutes, or as on one occasion, until Paddy Hurley stopped vomiting at the bow end of the boat. Then, the slow row back and the boat haul over the weir to the boathouse. Of course the race would be revisited that night over pints of stout. As the evening wore on, and certainly before the pub closed, we were convinced that in a day or two, a call would be received from the organizers of the fabled Henley Regatta in England, requesting our participation.

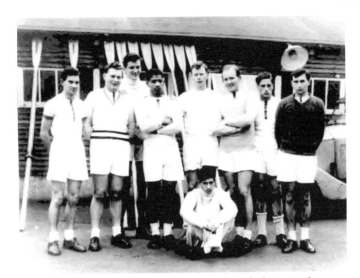

Third from Left, Pat O'Brien, Fourth from Left,
Hari Lamki, then Gene, Mike Thomas.
Seated Is Tim Meaghar, Team's Coxsman

Although I've highlighted the drudgery of the sport, there were times, especially when the wind was down and the Liffey glass-like, when it all came together. The boat balanced, a comfortable rhythm established, eight oars soundlessly striking the water as one, the lift of the bow - and doing it time and again on a crisp, sun-spent late afternoon was a beautiful thing.

University College Galway hosted an annual rowing event, and on my first foray into that part of the country our crew did well, coming in second to the host team and ahead of three local eights. We felt pretty good about ourselves as we headed home. The journey took us through the Irish mid-lands, a desolate topography: vast reaches of gray bog encircled by low-lying hills. White painted cottages, widely spaced, accented the gloom.

We stopped in a small village for a petrol fill-up. The attendant, a young man, was all a-chatter about a recent storm, and yes, we should be in Dublin in two hours but we "couldn't tarry along the way."

"What's the name of this town?" I asked.

"Cloghan," he answered.

Cloghan, Cloghan...that sounds familiar. Then the penny dropped - Dorcan. I turned to the others. "Hold on. Got to make a quick phone call. I know someone who lives around here. It'll only take a couple of minutes."

The glass of the kiosk door was broken, slivering the light as I looked through the phone book and found the number.

"Hello, is Seamus there?" I asked.

A female voice answered, "And who is this?"

"Gene McKee; I roomed with him on the Mauritania, a couple years ago."

"Oh, the young student. He talked about you. I'm his daughter, Moira." She hesitated. "My Dad's gone. He passed away awhile back."

"I'm sorry. What happened?"

"Had an accident with the lorry. Up on Byrne Head; went off the cliff and crashed into the rocks at the bottom." She paused. "No one could understand, with him knowing the roads so well."

"When?"

"Just after Grammy died. Became very quiet and to himself, just wasn't the same. But," she continued, "he often spoke of you, the young Yank. Both of you afraid to get off the boat."

"And he told me about you. I even know the color of your eyes."

There was a sniffle. "I didn't mind, you know?"

"Mind?" I asked.

"How he looked. He was still my handsome dad; I miss him terrible."

A horn was heard in the distance. "I've got to get going. I'm so sorry."

"Thanks, and thanks for calling. He was hoping you would one day. God Bless."

"Goodbye, Moira, and good luck."

Poor bastard. As I turned to leave I saw my face smudged

and distorted by the cracked glass of the kiosk door. *How weird, just like the mirror in the cabin.* The horn was more insistent as I ran toward the van.

Luckily, we did get to Dublin before the pubs closed.

Formal Events and the Tara Street Baths

The social highlights of the year were the two or three college-sponsored formal dances. Invitations were extended to all in the college with a good cross section in attendance. The events were held at either the Gresham or Shelbourne hotels. My preparation for these evenings included a tuxedo rental, a haircut, and on the afternoon of the event, a tub booked at the Tara Street Baths in Dublin. For the price of a half crown, you were assigned a small room which contained a large tub, on the side of which was draped a brown towel. Also included: a bar of gray-yellow soap, whose essential component (something akin to carbolic acid), left skin the texture of sandpaper; as a shampoo, hair loss had been reported. For an extra sixpence a scented bar was available, which for such an occasion I considered money well spent. Buoyed by an extravagant amount of hot water, I luxuriated in the womb-like warmth until my hands crinkled. Leaving Tara Street I was clean, wrinkled, smelling good, and ready for the night.

Accompanying women to these dances did not imply a romantic interest. They were classmates who wanted to attend and needed an escort. A good time was had but once the evening was over, it was over. The following day you reverted to classmate status. That was not to say that the occasional relationship never developed. There were two or three couples in our class, who in the parlance of the day, were "doing a line." But most relationships developed outside the college setting.

On one such occasion I escorted a very attractive woman - and a recently qualified physician - Delia McCartan, to her Conferring Ball at the Gresham Hotel. For a large part of the evening, I could be found drinking with the boys at a bar adjacent to the hotel - my rudeness knew no bounds in those days. When the evening ended, and in spite of my behavior, Delia invited me to her flat. Amazed and delighted, I figured the scented soap had finally kicked in.

"I have something for you," she said, "which I'm sure you'll enjoy."

A host of possibilities raced through my mind. "What?" I asked.

"You'll know soon enough."

Upon arrival at the flat, Delia put a record on the phonograph. Setting the mood, I assumed; how romantic, I thought. Quickly I slipped my bow tie into a jacket pocket and opened the top button of my shirt. I was ready!

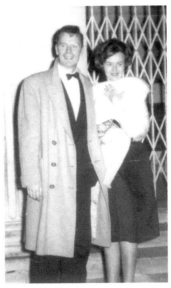

Gene with Delia McCartan - Conferring Ball
Gresham Hotel, December 1, 1960

The record turned out to be Beethoven's Sixth Symphony, the "Pastoral," which we proceeded to listen to in its entirety. At intervals I affirmed my appreciation. Delia said that she knew I would love it and was delighted that I had. Unfortunately, that was all Delia shared with me that night. Although my randy expectations were dashed, it was a fun time and she was right: that particular symphony has been a favorite of mine since; the enjoyment probably enhanced by my recollection of its introduction.

In the spring and on other occasions during the horse racing season, Pat O'Brien's father visited from England. His usual destination was the Curraugh in County Kildare, world-renown as a flat racing and horse training venue. On arrival in Dublin, he treated Pat and me to a meal at the Dolphin Hotel.

One of Dublin's more up-scale scenes, their food was considered the best in the city, especially their steaks. Appetites whetted by a pint or two of stout, we dined at the wide, polished mahogany bar. A male domain, seldom were women seen at the tables scattered about the rather formal lounge. Its ambiance boasted carpet, floor lamps, and somber wainscoting capped by dreary fawn-colored wallpaper, depicting equally dreary country scenes. The properly attired men at the tables involved in quiet conversation or immersed in their newspapers, seemed to be men of business; their drink of choice, in most instances, was whiskey with a side of water.

"Yes, it should be a grand season," Dr. O'Brien continued as we discussed the upcoming Cup event. "The greatest horses in the world are coming to Ireland these days. Gene, have you ever heard of Vincent O'Brien?" he asked. "No relation," he added.

"Just the name, Doctor; I know he's in racing."

"Well, he trains horses and he's put this country on the map. Extraordinary success, both on the flat and steeplechase."

"His horse won the Grand National a few years ago," chimed in Pat. "More than once, I think."

His father nodded. "Three times, three consecutive years and with three different horses!"

The conversation veered to other topics (school being one which Pat and I tiptoed around) as we enjoyed our meal.

I remember mine well: a large, medium-rare steak, juices oozing, accompanied by a tower of whipped, creamed potatoes with a side of soft, fried onions. Dessert followed: warm apple pie and ice cream, or if available, warm tapioca pudding submerged in pour cream. Always a great night out and a welcome respite from the digs' fare.

(The Dolphin Hotel is no longer, but the memories of my visits are still relished.)

An Afternoon with Joe

With a more relaxed schedule that spring, I became friendly with the mystery man of Hyde House, Miss Halligan's nephew. Joe worked second shift and was seldom seen during the day. Passing his room on the way to breakfast, I often heard the rustle of newspapers and a hard cigarette cough.

In his mid-to-late 40's, Joe was tall and pale complexioned, with acne scars on both cheeks. Always well-groomed, with coat, tie, and polished black shoes, his pomaded black hair, long in the back, curled over a white shirt collar.

Joe worked for *The Irish Times*, employed there since coming to Dublin some fifteen years prior. Beginning as a linotype operator he had progressed to his present position, proofreader for the morning edition. Like many in that profession, Joe liked his drink.

On a couple of occasions Joe asked me to join him for lunch. Typically, we began around noon at a pub off Synge Street. At this hour, Joe was shaky, face a pasty white, voice tremulous, even his gait seemed out of synch. The bar had a skittles table, a game Joe enjoyed, and in which he was proficient. Setting the pins on the table, inserting a coin to activate the game or even lighting a cigarette, required his full concentration. However, after a pint or two with a side of whiskey, color returned, tremor resolved, and he was fine for the remainder of the day. I, on the other hand, well out of my drinking league, nursed bottles of stout through the afternoon.

Working our way into the city, we stopped at pubs along Camden Street where Joe was a regular. We had a mid-afternoon lunch of sandwiches and hard boiled eggs. Conversations with Joe were never extensive. He spoke in a jerky rhythm, sentences short, as if anxious to get them over with and move along to other things. Eschewing interest in Ireland's history he offered no pretense of curiosity in its arts, politics or sports. While he knew which play was at the Gate or Gaiety theatres, was able to tick off soccer scores, hurling results, and the critiques of Brendan Behan's latest effort, his knowledge didn't extend beyond what he proofread in the newspaper. For the listener, it was similar to hearing news clips on the radio.

As we chatted and finished our lunch - the tab for which Joe picked up - I was struck by how constricted and unfulfilling his life seemed, at least to me. What we did that afternoon was what Joe did every afternoon, along with a work shift that effectively negated any nighttime activities. Probably in his late forties, Joe presented a fine appearance: tall, no extra weight, well dressed, intelligent, with decent looks. He would have had little problem finding one of the fairer sex to spend some time with and perhaps expand his horizon. Yet he evinced little interest in anything be-yond his usual routine. My comment: "Fine looking chap like you, Joe, should get himself a girlfriend," merely provoked a quick smile and the reply: "Don't have time for that stuff." Then he shifted conversation to another subject. Probably of greater concern to Joe, in the not-too-distant future, would be his liver.

Eventually we got to Joe's turf, the pubs along the quays of the Liffey River. *The Irish Times* was located in the area so we stayed in the vicinity until it was time for Joe to report for work. Near O'Connell Bridge, pub patrons were a mixed bag: business people, laborers and the occasional student. Farther down river were the bars that served the dock workers and those off the boats. Seldom was a woman or mixed drink seen. Hard-working and hard-looking men, theirs was not the noisy camaraderie of the pubs nearer the city. Their work finished, they took their pints at the bar or engaged in conversation at tables around a small lounge filled with smoke and the smell of their sweat.

Joe was involved in a local skittles league where the com-petition was intense. On occasion I played as his partner and although a good player myself, I was clearly outmatched. Not only an excellent competitor, but of equal merit in that crowd, was Joe's ability to return, as quickly as received, the volley of banter that accompanied each shot.

After that spring I saw Joe only occasionally, and when I left Dublin he was still in the digs. (Some years later, on a trip to Ireland, Miss Halligan informed me he was home and not well.)

That summer I returned home to replenish the financial coffers – hopefully saving enough to finance another year in Ireland. As usual, the fish and I met at the co-op six days a week; Fridays I caddied for my spending money. Bertha and my father were pleased with my progress. They expressed cautious optimism that the plan for medical school which had begun, to use an American football analogy, as a Hail Mary pass, might yet be successful.

The sacrifices that Bertha made for me during these years was seldom acknowledged. Besides her persistence and enthusiasm, she provided the necessary funding. My aunt covered all tuition shortfalls; every month for six years, she sent a check for room and board. Ship passages and a trip through Europe were part of her largesse. The things she did without, the vacations not taken - so I could go to school - was an exceptional generosity, the benefits of which have lasted a lifetime.

About a week before I was scheduled to leave for Ireland, a large packet arrived from Cunard with my ticket, boarding details, baggage tags, and some health precaution hand-outs.

As was her habit, Bertha read anything she felt pertinent out loud to me.

"Just think, Bert, this will be the last time you'll be doing this."

She smiled. "Hopefully."

I hesitated, then spoke quickly. "I appreciate all you've done for me. I hope you know that."

"It'll be worth it, if you make it." She looked over at me. "And someday when you're rich and famous, you can give me a trip."

"Anywhere you want. Anywhere. Just name it."

"How about around the world? Can you handle that?"

"I'm not kidding, Bert."

She smiled; there was a twinkle in her eye. "I'm not either."

"Whatever, I just wanted to thank you, that's all."

"It's OK, Gene. Don't be so serious."

I went to give her a hug, but she had turned away before I got there.

I also visited my mother before I left. She was pleased that I was doing well and promised, if not material support, to keep me in her prayers. (It was only decades later, my mother immersed and delighted in her grandmother role, that I became aware of, and felt badly about, the years of our detachment: how little attention I had paid her and how empty her life. Now when she visited, not only were my kids getting to know her, I was also. One can't rewind the tapes and edit the past, but it can be said in truth, that when her story ended, she had found her son and he, his mother.)

The *Mauritania* was again booked for my return to Ireland. To my surprise, Tom Conneen was a fellow passenger, seemingly more laid-back and relaxed. No invitations to socialize with the young ladies in first class were forthcoming this trip, but we didn't lack for things to keep us occupied.

The third day into the trip the weather changed, and placid waters became storm-swept; torrents of wind-driven rain lashed the vessel. All outside activities on the ship were cancelled. Most passengers, many who became quite seasick, hunkered down in their cabins to wait it out.

It so happened that I was involved in a ping-pong tournament. About six of the fifteen or so passengers that had entered the competition remained. Arriving at the area where the matches took place, only two people were present: a crew member and a young boy (twelve-years-old, I later learned). His left arm was casted and in a sling; fortunately he was right-handed.

After waiting a few more minutes, the crew member said, "I guess no one else is coming, and probably won't in this weather.

Why don't you two play and whoever wins can claim the championship trophy?" He took a small (probably eight inch), statuette from a box - a replica of the *Mauretania* - and placed it face down on a table, then left the room.

The match began - a two-out-of-three-game series - and this red-headed kid was good, real good. Everything I hit at him he rocketed back in spades. As the ship pitched and bucked through the heavy seas it was increasingly difficult to maintain footing. For the youngster it was especially treacherous: weighing no more than ninety pounds, he was flung back and forth, unable to use his left arm for balance. Several times when he reached for a shot his casted arm fell out of the sling and he frantically tried to re-insert it while playing. Seizing the advantage, hungry for victory, I smashed the ball, time and again, past his dangling limb. But he hung in there, forcing a third game. *No quit in this one*, I thought. However, with the worsening weather conditions and the frequent sling malfunctions, I eventually out-slugged him and eked out a victory.

I went to him and put out my hand. "Good match, young fellow."

He looked at me, lower lip quivering, eyes starting to fill. Abruptly he turned and ran from the room. His sobs could be heard echoing down the corridor.

And there I stood, fondling my trophy; savoring the achievement. A tug of compassion surfaced as I thought of the little tyke, probably crying inconsolably in his mother's arms. But the tug passed quickly. "Probably did the lad a good turn," I reasoned. "A lesson for life: can't win 'em all." Generous, as one should be in victory, I acknowledged that the youngster put up a good fight. "And he'll be back one day; the kid's a comer," I said to myself.

Clutching my trophy and with a bit of a cockiness in my step, I went off to find Tom. (An addendum will be noted later.)

The morning of our fifth day at sea, a verdant landscape appeared on the horizon and shortly after, the cathedral spire at Cobh was sighted. Tom and I soon disembarked, cleared Customs, bussed to Cork and within an hour were seated on the train to Dublin.

Miss Halligan welcomed me back and informed me that the core group: Joe, Frank, Lorna and Dan remained intact. Also, at least for the present, I would have a room to myself. Settling in, I felt happy to be back and looked forward to the new school year: subjects more directly related to medicine. It would be my first experience in a hospital setting, and hopefully I would come upon something able to provoke an interest in a field which so far had been found lacking.

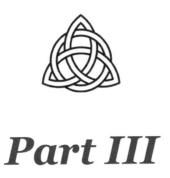

Part III

A few faces were missing as our class gathered for the new school year – victims of the "half" exam. For them, the acquisition of a stethoscope – the totem of prestige and achievement that signaled your "arrival" in clinical medicine – was placed on hold. My purchase was made at a surgical supply house on Grafton St. Seen about town, with the ear pieces discretely peeking from your jacket pocket, was the ultimate status symbol, a not too subtle acknowledgment of your membership in the medical school hierarchy.

It also symbolized the transition between the didactics of the pre-clinical years – the abstractions of the sciences, the mind-numbing memorizations of anatomy, the complexities of physiology – to their application to real people, books to bodies. The overture had been played, the real action was about to commence. So in spite of myself, I noticed a smidgen of seriousness had been acquired.

The next year, I felt, would be decisive: any affinity I might have for the practice of medicine, or lack thereof, would become apparent. Though I had achieved a measure of success to that point, nothing was a game-changer. My doubts and lack of interest were as real as ever, but the good time I was having provided on-going compensation. Almost as an outside observer, I was curious as to what the outcome might be.

Medicine, as an art, rather than a science, was demonstrated daily in the teaching hospitals of that era. The technological avalanche, soon to arrive, was but a sail breeching a distant horizon. The only diagnostic modalities available were x-rays, cardiograms and a limited spectrum of lab tests. Accurate diagnosis was directly related to the skill of the physician.

A vast literature existed, dedicated solely to the clinical signs associated with various disease states. In the pulmonary area, for example, breath sounds were described as either vesicular or tubular; rhonchi: sonorous or sibilant. Lung consolidations, demonstrated by percussion, were further defined by the absence or presence of bronchophony or whispered pectoriloquy. Such distinctions identified the underlying pathology and the probable diagnosis.

As neophytes, such skills were yet to be realized. But exposed to that level of clinical acumen, we became reasonably adept. Our daily tasks were more pedestrian. We made rounds, practiced our history-taking skills, participated in physical examinations, performed minor lab tests, and did what the floor nurses told us. At Mercer's Hospital I observed my first major surgery, a gastrectomy performed by Mr. Matthews. (The prefix Dr. was replaced by Mr. when fellowship had been attained, analogous to board certification in the United States.)

I came to enjoy the patient's story: how the illness presented, the past, and family histories. Once the required sections of the medical record had been completed, I often stayed and chatted with the patient. Small talk, unrelated to their illness, ranged from sports to politics. My accent invariably brought the United States into the conversation, and without exception, each patient had a connection to the country, either through relatives or a trip taken. Mention of Dublin as my mother's birthplace or my grandfather's emigration ("From County Tyrone, was he now?"), elicited torrents of recollection and questions. By the end of the chat, to which I contributed little, it was definitely established that the patient and I were within shouting distance of being third cousins. Everyone has a story to tell and no one tells theirs better than the Irish, real or imagined; it was a fun part of the job.

The down-side occurred when the patient, now a friend, had a bad outcome and their misfortune, which otherwise wouldn't warrant a second thought, acquired a personal dimension. Even at that stage I came to realize the merit of not getting too close to patients; be friendly, yes, but at a distance. (Learned later and equally true: Never go to a patient's wake. Being introduced as "the doctor who took care of Daddy," now lying stiff and stark in the box a few feet away, is never a good thing especially in a small town.)

Mr. Bouchier-Hayes was Chief of Surgery at Mercer's at the time and something of a legend relative to his surgical accomplishments. My personal anecdote regarding Mr. Hayes occurred while making rounds with him one morning. Overseeing my examination of an abdomen, he noted my nicotine-stained fingers, high-lighted against the white skin of the patient. Stopping the examination, he said: "You'll not be back until your hands are clean," and he dismissed me from the group. It was then that I became acquainted with the pumice stone.

(Over the years, I have come to appreciate more fully the clinical skills of the physicians I encountered at Mercer's and other hospitals during my years in Dublin. Today's diagnoses by MRI's, CT scans, and a host of other radiological and lab technologies, were made by clinicians using only their hands, eyes, and minds. Sadly, in the spirit of full disclosure and malpractice concerns, I count myself among the present day crop.)

Jervis Street Hospital

Early that first year, I decided to leave Mercer's and transfer to the Jervis Street Hospital, Dublin's largest inner city facility, run by the Sisters of Mercy. Mercer's offered excellent teaching, but being relatively small, did not have the volume and variety of pathology found at the larger institution. Jervis Street, a sturdy, square of a building, was located just up from Bachelor's Walk and the Liffey River and aside from some scrolling along the fourth floor cornice, offered little architectural pretense. Originally a mansion for one of the English gentry, it was converted to a hospital in the early 1800s. Through its doors flowed the most woebegone of Dublin's ill and injured. For the student, it seemed like the place to be. (As an historical aside, many of those injured in the 1916 Easter Uprising, centered a few blocks away on O'Connell Street, were brought there for treatment.)

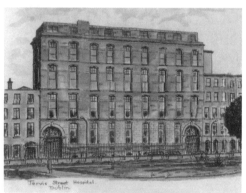

Jervis Street Hospital

The emergency room, especially busy on Friday and weekend nights, accounted for roughly 75% of the hospital's admissions. Patients with a variety of injuries, often associated with a degree of intoxication, presented regularly. I learned to suture there, the doctor on duty delighted for the help. Local anesthesia was available but often not needed. The procedure finished, the patient was usually complimentary: "Ah sure, but you're a fine young doctor." Hopefully those sentiments remained intact when one's handiwork was viewed the following morning.

Soon after we started third year, Tom Lomas and I decided to share a flat. We felt it offered a better place to study, and more to the point, would provide a place to bring the women - whom surely we would find - eager for seduction. With some guilt, I told Miss Halligan I had an in-hospital residency requirement and would return to the digs when finished. She said she would hold a room for me.

A place was found on lower Rathmines Road and it worked out well. Tom was easy to live with - much more focused on things academic than I - a positive influence. The rent was slightly more than expected but that was balanced by a frugal life-style. Food was purchased at a small shop across the street. Breakfast consisted of bread, a couple of eggs and a pint of milk; a potato or two with some form of meat comprised our evening meal. Lunch we ate at the college. In the apartment, food expenditures were about three shillings a day, fifty cents in American money. Hard to believe in retrospect, but the purchase of one potato, a single tomato, four Brussels sprouts, a slice of meat, or just two cigarettes was not unusual; many others did the same.

The demise of our co-habitation came about in an interesting way. Preparation for the Materia Medica (pharmacology) exam was our primary academic focus at the time: a major test which, if failed, would be a significant setback. Tom and I put in an adequate amount of study, but because of the importance and difficulty of the exam, we felt we should be doing more. At the end of a long day, however, it was increasingly difficult to stay awake much beyond 10:00 p.m.

Sarah Killian (name altered), a final-year pharmacology student at UCD and I were keeping company at the time. Sarah also worked part-time at a chemist shop in Dublin. Mentioning our fatigue situation, she said she could help. The label, Dexedrine, was affixed to the bottle of pills she provided. "They're guaranteed to maintain alertness," she said. This was long before amphetamines and speed entered the popular culture.

Tom and I used the medication, and as advertised, the effect was immediate and extraordinary; additionally, we both noted a sense of well-being and an increased confidence in our ability to understand and retain the material. With one pill, or occasionally two, we were good for most of the night. Prior to the exam we were studying four to five hours a day, attending class, hospital rounds and clinics, while remaining remarkably alert.

The morning of the exam the medication wasn't used; we felt it had done its job. The exam questions, after a quick perusal, seemed straight forward and not particularly difficult. A wisp of concern surfaced when I couldn't remember my student ID number (6122), requested on the answer booklet. "No problem," I said to myself, "it will come to me later." When pen was put to paper the questions that seemed so routine initially, were now as indecipherable as a foreign language. Then began the nausea and sweating: my clothes stuck to me. Totally strung out and unable to summon any semblance of recall, I wrote a few sentences for each question and left.

Tom went through a similar experience. We both failed the exam, which at that time, felt catastrophic. Probably at the insistence of his family, Tom moved out of the flat, to the opposite side of the city, and I rejoined Miss Halligan. We parted as friends and remained friends, certainly wiser for the experience. So the apartment experiment ended - actually a good time - and although the anticipated deluge of wild women didn't materialize, we did have our moments.

The relationship with Sarah continued: a liaison that began one night at a party when a tall, attractive, well put together woman asked if I was a medical student.

"I am; but don't hold it against me," I replied. "Just a phase I'm going through."

She laughed. "Until you grow up, right?"

"Exactly." *Pretty quick comeback*, I thought.

"That's what I want to do."

"So why don't you?"

Her family, she explained, owned a chemist shop and since, of her siblings, she had achieved the best grades in school, she was designated to continue the tradition, the third generation. "I'm doing pharmacology and will finish in about a year. It's alright," she continued, "but if I had my druthers, I'd do medicine. How about you; do you like it?"

"Family pressure is part of my story," I told her. And with this as background, we chatted back and forth for a good portion of the evening.

Whether it was the interesting conversation or her well-proportioned body that prompted me to ask for a phone number, I don't recollect. A few days later I inserted three pennies into a phone box and dialed the number; she agreed it would be fun to get together.

An art exhibit would not have been my choice for our meeting, but she thought it an appropriate place for me to "bump into her." After some desultory conversation and shared observations relative to a series of repetitive Irish landscapes, Sarah said she would meet me outside the art house. During the walk to her place near Merrion Square, she explained her somewhat aloof behavior at the exhibit. Though not formerly engaged, she was very involved with a man near her home and was hesitant to be seen with another male lest it find its way back to him. A wedding was planned after she obtained her degree.

Graciously acceding to her wish not to be seen in public, I would visit after the pubs closed. Her bed-sitter consisted of a small kitchenette, bathroom, and a bed that usurped most of the remaining space. Sarah was curious, intelligent, and conversant in a variety of subjects, all leavened with a terrific sense of humor. After a drink or two and a bite to eat we listened to the wireless (Radio Luxembourg's Top Twenty tunes on Sunday nights), socialized, and sometime later I headed home.

This arrangement lasted, intermittently, for her remaining time in Dublin. While doing my clerkship at the Rotunda Hospital, I received a letter indicating that she had passed her exams and was returning home. So ended our relationship; the compatibility was such that at another time and under different circumstances we might have taken a more serious turn.

(Many years later, in 1981, the McKee family toured Ireland. Passing through her hometown, I stopped at her family's chemist shop. Sarah was not there, but her brother happened to be in the shop. Sarah, he informed me, was happily married with four children. In the note I left I wished her well and hoped that a few memories remained of the good times we had in Dublin those many years ago.)

Although not in frequent touch with Tom Conneen at Trinity, occasionally we'd meet at a party or social event. As a result, I met some of his friends, who in turn, were introduced to the mainstays of my set. Colin Condron, a classmate of Tom's, and a dead ringer for Gordon McRae, the movie actor, became an acquaintance. Relationships developed to the extent that four or five of us were invited to his home in England for a few days during the upcoming Christmas holidays. Colin was from Blackpool, a popular vacation resort in County Lancashire on England's west coast. His father and mother ran a rooming house, catering to the influx of tourists in the summer, so ample lodging was available off-season. Colin's father also managed the local golf course.

Colin's parents were extraordinarily accommodating to our unruly, but appreciative, group. Weather permitting, we played golf daily and partied nights. The availability of empty rooms proved to be a distinct social benefit.

New Year's Eve was a special occasion. After midnight was struck and "Auld Lang Syne" rendered, we headed to the street to join other revelers and trekked through the neighborhood, all in great voice. Stops were made at various homes, and the occupants were serenaded; in most instances, this resulted in an invitation to enter the house. After we toasted the landlord, wished his family an abundance of blessings for the New Year, we left a small bag of coal and exited out the back door and onto the next home. The significance of the ritual was lost on me, but it was all great fun.

Colin's hospitality was accepted three or four times over the remaining years in Dublin (including his coming-of-age party), and we were never disappointed. The purported reserve and aloofness of the English was never my experience. Some older gentlemen, however, still harbored grudges toward the Yanks:

specifically those who after WW II brought all the good-looking women in England back to the States. The typical Irish riposte: "They wouldn't have needed a very big boat."

A Father-Son Road Trip

Hinted at, but thought unlikely, my father visited me during the summer of my third medical school year. His trip manifested a couple of firsts and a long-standing wish: first trip outside the United States, first trip on a transatlantic-liner, and Ireland at last. My concerns as I waited dockside for his arrival were two-fold: that he didn't have an enjoyable crossing and would want to take the next boat back, and secondly, he would become bored during our two week-long trip.

My father, to say the least, was not a social animal – other than being a member of the Knights of Columbus (pretty much insisted on by his father, a Fourth Degree member) – he belonged to no organizations. Aside from a Christmas get-together at work, there were no outside parties, no one visited at home, nor do I ever recollect him receiving a social phone call. There were no male or female companions. His one vice was playing the horses and once a year, on his vacation, he headed to Florida and the Hialeah racetrack, staying in the same rooming house on each visit. Bertha, on occasion, had a party in the house. Often he attended, but just as often, when the sociability requirements became uncomfortable, he left. I could imagine him being ill at ease in the pervasively convivial atmosphere aboard ship.

Apart from two cruises (three-day packages from Providence, on the Colonial Line, to New York City, where we ate at the Automat and went to the Roxy theater), my dad and I had never travelled together. My goal for this trip was to give him a good time – an experience to remember – and I worried whether I could accomplish this.

The man who disembarked at Cobh couldn't wait to tell me of the wonderful crossing he experienced: the great food, the fun group at his table each night (he had photos of them), the farewell party, great weather, and on and on. He actually had addresses of people to contact when he arrived home. I couldn't have been more pleased - shocked - but definitely pleased.

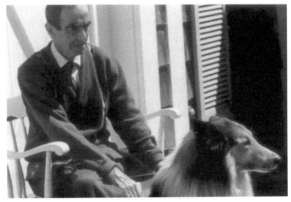

Gene's Dad and Kerry

The next day we toured the Cork area and then pushed on to Dublin.

Miss Halligan was delighted to meet him and had nothing but nice things to say about his son. Dublin's highlights were visited and a photograph taken of us at McKee Barracks, an Irish Army training center.

A slight upset occurred when I departed the digs one evening to purchase an extra pack of cigarettes, bumped into a friend, Freda Blaney, and didn't return until about 1:00 a.m. When I did arrive back he was awake and justifiably upset with me. My father's temper was more silent than violent. A good screaming match provides the material for a decent row. That was not my father's style.

"You knew I'd be worried," he began. There were about a half dozen cigarette butts in the ashtray.

"Totally thoughtless, Dad. I'm sorry. Just wasn't aware of the time."

His relief was obvious, but the concern tumbled out. "You could have had an accident. I wondered if I should go to the police. Even thought of waking Miss Halligan." He looked at me quickly, then turned away; perhaps he wished to maintain the scolding tone and not give way to emotion after hours of worry.

"It won't happen again, Dad. I promise. Let's get some sleep."

"I hope not."

He got into his bed, said goodnight and turned off the bedside light. The incident wasn't mentioned again.

My dad wanted to see something of the north of Ireland - his father was from County Tyrone. The original plan was to visit there, but we didn't know the exact name of the village of his birth or names of relatives that might help us. Researching our family heritage was never a priority in the McKee household. I had an interest, but repeated questions over the years elicited little information. The only things I knew of my grandfather was that he left Ireland in the 1870s, couldn't read or write, never went on a boat again after his trip to America, and worked at the textile mills in Pawtucket, R.I. for nine dollars a week. A similar dearth of information also applied to my mother's family.

We took a train to Belfast. After a night's rest, we rented a car and, deciding against County Tyrone, drove through beautiful countryside as far west as Donegal, an area of Ireland as new to me as him. Over two days, without a particular itinerary, we followed the coastline south from Donegal Bay to Sligo; a more picturesque drive you can't imagine. The bed and breakfasts: clean, comfortable, and casual, suited my father's preference in lodging perfectly.

Nervous that my dad would be antsy to return home or unable to tolerate the exigencies that come with touring without a fixed schedule or reservations in hand, proved to be needless. Much to my surprise and delight, he exhibited patience with the minor mishaps one expects in travel and a sociability I'd seldom seen and never expected. After our two-day sojourn along the coast, seeing his response to what would be a primer for the remainder of the trip, I knew that we would be fine together. He seemed totally comfortable in his tourist role.

Back in Dublin we booked passage on the B&I steamer and after crossing a surprisingly tranquil Irish Sea to Liverpool, made our way to London. More frugal than I, my father vetoed a couple of my "high class" room choices, favoring instead a truly crummy boarding house in a run-down section of town. But I managed to show him many of the tourist attractions in the city, accomplished, of course, on foot. My father wasn't too impressed with London for some reason, probably because he felt it wasn't appropriate for an Irishman to enjoy anything English.

After London we went to Paris and stayed at my old digs in Val d'Or. Father Wright still maintained his residence there, but at the time of our arrival, was on holiday. The boarders of my recollection had long gone. The local families that had befriended me during my earlier stay remained, were glad to see me, and were especially nice to my dad, which I appreciated. My father was impressed with my French facility.

Courtesy of Grey Line, we toured Paris and visited its main attractions. The oppressive humidity had taken its toll on my father, which allowed this extravagance. With a rented car at our disposal, we spent a day at Versailles followed by a drive to Chartres, the site of the oldest and most famous medieval cathedral in France.

My father, as a young man, spent two years in a seminary of the LaSallette Order preparing to become a priest. For reasons never revealed, he dropped out (much to the displeasure, Bertha indicated, of his mother and father). His devotion to the church never faltered, and he was always impressed with anything portraying the grandeur and glory of the Church, and the cathedral at Chartres would have it all. The trip, about fifty miles, took us through broad reaches of wheat fields, interrupted by the occasional vineyard. Soon a church spire pierced the distant horizon and phoenix-like the cathedral slowly emerged - the structure so imposing, we were hardly aware of the picturesque village that surrounded it.

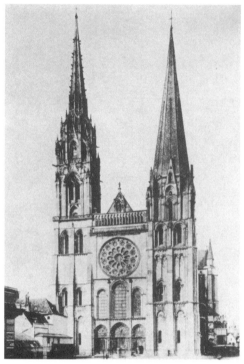

Chartres Cathedral

Considered the finest example of French Gothic architecture, construction began in 1194 and was completed 160 years later. Incredibly, the cathedral survived not only the ravages and tantrums of time, but the French Revolution and WW II. At one point during this latter conflict, the cathedral was suspected to be headquarters for German operations in the area, and as such, targeted for destruction by American guns. On hearing this, an intrepid American colonel requested and received permission to covertly determine if the cathedral was, in fact, being used by the enemy. He reported back that it was unoccupied, the proposed bombardment was cancelled, and the cathedral was spared. The same colonel was killed a few weeks later.

The interior was impressive: a vast nave with clustered columns that supported a curved ceiling hundreds of feet above, side altars sculpted with intricate design. Centuries old, stained-glass windows splashed vivid color across the tiled floor. Scattered amongst the aisles people knelt in prayer; guides passed by leading their small groups.

In that vast and holy space we found a pew, and as centuries of souls had before us, offered an Ave or two. Certain settings exposed sentimentality in my dad: a choir singing "Silent Night" on Christmas Eve, news reels relating to domestic tragedies, Kate Smith singing "God Bless America." And so it was that afternoon in the solemnity and majesty of Chartres when I became aware of his small coughs and the occasional handkerchief dab to his face. Without glancing, I knew there were tears in his eyes. Re-thinking the episode some days later, I wondered if the emotion was in response to the magnificent edifice surrounding us, or rather, the memory of his lost vocation. (Years later he still spoke of that visit.)

From France we re-traced our steps to England, Ireland, and Cobh where my father boarded the ship for home. He told me that the trip was one of the nicest times he had ever had in his life. Whether or not my aunt Bertha told him to say that when the visit ended, I don't know. I took him at his word and was glad I was able to give some pleasure to a man whom I don't think had an abundance of that commodity in his day.

That same summer, after Pathology was passed, I began a two-month, clinical clerkship at Jervis Street. Before beginning the final year and sitting exams in Medicine and Surgery, the college handbook stated: "A student must do six months as a surgical dresser and six months as a medical dresser." This basically meant attaching yourself to one or more of the consultants in each discipline for the prescribed time; it was also recommended that a portion of that time include residence in a hospital, which I would accomplish with the clerkship.

Apart from the in-hospital experience there were other advantages: excellent food with a varied menu, no rent payment (so extra money), an opportunity to check out the nurses, and in newly constructed living quarters, my own room which contained the greatest luxury of all - a shower.

My position as a cellar-dweller in the hospital hierarchy was to be expected, being one of the rookies. On the top tier reigned the physician consultant, either medical or surgical. To my knowledge there were no female medical or surgical consultants at Jervis Street at that time. Next in line were the registrars, senior or junior, dependent on their experience level - comparable to a resident in American hospitals. In most cases, they were physicians preparing for membership or fellowship in either medicine or surgery. Beneath them were the interns and finally the students (clerks). Once assigned, the student participated in the history-taking and medical examinations of in-patients, attended out-patient clinics, and worked in the Emergency Room.

During this period - almost a year into the clinical medicine scene - an awareness developed: I was enjoying my medical school situation. No burning bush epiphany or sudden realization that I had found my life's calling, but rather a cautious optimism that maybe this medicine business might be O.K. On occasion, in the company of students in other disciplines - engineering, law, business, the classics - I'd ask myself if I would trade my situation for theirs. Invariably the answer was "no." And that told me something. Plus, I thought the medical students livelier, less constricted in their thinking, with an unexpected propensity for outlandish behavior. "Oh, he's just one of those crazy medical students..." was often the rationalization offered at such times. And being in medicine we had the mystique that would never be theirs.

The key, I realized, was my introduction to the hospital. Early on in this new environment, patient rounds in the morning offered a glimpse of academics transposed to the bedside. When the attending and his retinue gathered around a patient - although much of the lab data and terminology bandied about was largely indecipherable to me - it was fun to listen to their opinions and interpretations as they put the elements of a diagnosis or treatment together. Students might be called on to comment regarding a case but generally they hovered, observed, and listened in the background. Seen but not heard would be an apt description. At that point, at the edge of the pack, I had little to offer other than my attention and an admiration for those with the abilities to make sense of it all (and hopefully help the poor bastard lying in the bed). Thus my interest was piqued. I wanted to be involved in the conversation.

Medical outpatient clinics began after morning rounds. Each patient was prepared for examination by a nurse who gathered pertinent background information and recent lab and x-ray data which were presented to the physician upon his arrival in the exam room. The student was meant to pay attention to the physician's comments and observations.

I was assigned to Dr. William Dwyer, a medical attending, who proved to be affable, knowledgeable, and unlike others, allowed student participation during patient exams. The clinic started at 8:00 a.m., with patients seen at fifteen minute intervals throughout the morning. Precisely at ten o'clock the schedule was interrupted for the mid-morning tea break. Tea pots, cloaked in warmers and accompanied by scones and an assortment of muffins, became available at a large table covered with a white tablecloth in the main office area. Dr. Dwyer was served an assortment of pastries and a pot of tea at his desk. Similar scenarios were enacted in all areas of the hospital, except perhaps the operating rooms. But even there it seemed more than happenstance that many surgical closures seemed to coincide with this mid-morning ritual.

The surgical rotation had a more irregular schedule with rounds accomplished either before or after the day's surgery with out-patient clinics often held in the afternoons. Students were allowed in the operating room with no specific role other than to observe, unless the surgeon made a different determination. Still, breaks were looked forward to and above the operating theater was a small room where students, interns, and nurses congregated between cases for tea and cigarettes. The cramped quarters provided opportunities for knee-to-knee conversations and benign flirting with the nurses. There I met Bernie Lavelle, a student nurse, with whom I later became quite friendly.

Mr. Walsh, a general surgeon with a sub-specialty in urology, provided my introduction to the surgical world. "Knocky" had a reputation for considering students a penance to be endured in return for surgical privileges at the hospital, along with being arrogant and difficult to work with. Part of his specialty training had been accomplished in the United States, a country he enjoyed, where he was treated well. Whether my nationality influenced the dynamic of our relationship, I don't know, but on rounds he often asked if I understood a particular aspect of the case under discussion. Occasionally he allowed me to assist at surgery. So mine was a positive experience, and while working with him, I met Nora.

"Always consider tuberculosis, Gentlemen," intoned Mr. Walsh to those huddled around him at the entrance to the third floor ward. Our group included the surgical registrar, an intern, me, and another medical student. Morning rounds were in progress prior to the day's surgeries.

"Began with the famine...," he continued, "...scratching for bits to eat, living like animals, and all the while, lorries packed with food, lumbered on their way to England."

Knocky Walsh looked and sounded as one would imagine a surgeon of some eminence. Tall, lean, patrician in appearance, he presented a clean-shaven, angular face, more distinguished than handsome, with carefully managed black hair. With thumbs hooked into his vest pockets, he spoke as of the manor born, with an accent that might be thought English, if not betrayed, on occasion, by his County Sligo roots.

Eye contact with Knocky was fleeting, his gaze fixed on some distant horizon. If in good humor, he allowed questions, but in most instances, his answer so caustically demonstrated the ineptitude of the questioner, the humiliation seemed hardly worth the additional information. His persona notwithstanding, no one questioned his surgical abilities.

"Today it's not the English," he continued, "but the miserable conditions the poor of this country live in...worse than the famine." Shaking his head he turned toward the door. "So let's visit our new arrival, shall we, Gentlemen?"

The patient was at the far end of a mixed medical/surgical ward. A blanket was pulled to her chin; her silhouette, framed by a fan of black hair, was distinguished by high cheekbones, an upturned nose and full lips. On our approach she turned. Her face, narrowed by a hint of gauntness, was by any definition, beautiful. The group halted at the foot of her bed.

"Good morning, Dear. I'm Mr. Walsh." He glanced at the clipboard at the end of the bed. "And you must be Nora?"

"Yes, sir."

"These," he gestured toward us, "are my assistants."

Nora nodded and briefly glanced in our direction. Carefully adjusting the pleat in his trousers, Mr. Walsh sat on the edge of the bed.

"Getting right to it, Nora, you know why you're here, do you not?"

"Yes, sir," she answered, without hesitation. "There's tuberculosis in me kidney. It don't work anymore, and it's got to be removed, before it spreads someplace else." Her speech was of Dublin city, short, rough phrases, without lilt or inflection.

"Yes, Nora, that's exactly right."

Mr. Walsh turned to the group. "Gentlemen, removal of the kidney is imperative for a number of reasons, but primarily, as Nora said, to prevent spread." Knocky, in his most professorial manner, then gave a brief overview of the pathology, the anatomy of the area, the surgical options, and the prognosis associated with the diagnosis. "Of course," he continued, "she'll need laboratory tests done and a medical examination before surgery, but such a young woman should be otherwise healthy."

Nora, very quiet up to this point, interrupted. "Begging your pardon, sir, but I do feel a proper fool, being looked up and down and talked about, with me having no say in the matter. I'm to be examined by the lot of ya, is it?"

"Well, Nora, you are on the service, you know."

"So it's a feckin' guinea pig, I am?"

"I suppose in a way you are, Nora," Knocky answered with a smile.

"Well," Nora replied, nodding toward the group, "will all of these be taking care of me or will I have a personal one?"

Mr. Walsh looked at the registrar. "Who has the exams this week?"

The registrar pointed to me. I raised my hand.

"Nora, this student will take your history, do an exam and present your case to the group. Everything, of course, will be re-checked by the registrar and if anything is amiss I will certainly be notified.

"Well," she replied, "he wouldn't have been me first choice, but I guess he'll do."

When I returned after the morning surgery, Nora was sitting on her bed, drying her hair.

"So, you're me doctor."

I shook my head. "I'm not a Doctor, just a student, like Mr. Walsh said."

"So what'll I call ya?"

Before I could answer, she added, "With an accent like that, you must be a Yank."

"Guilty."

Wrapping her towel turban-style around her head, she said, "Then Yank it will be."

I took her history the following morning. Before I began I mentioned that to properly complete the medical record, I needed to ask some personal questions. "I'm not trying to pry into your private life," I added.

"Ask anything you like," she replied.

Every question was answered directly; she was twenty-four-years-old and single. "I'm not that daft ya know." She was named after Nora Barnacle, "someone in a book me ma read." Inquiring into her family history, she indicated she was the old-est of three children; the others, a boy and a girl, were twelve and fourteen years of age respectively. Her father only did odd jobs because "of a problem" while her mother operated a vege-table and fruit cart on Camden Street. "Not to brag," she said, "but I was very smart in me studies." She felt badly she hadn't finished secondary school. Presently employed at the Jacobs Biscuit Factory, she worked second shift, earning seven pounds a week. Her preference was first shift but she had to care for the younger kids during the day.

This was her first time in hospital. She said it started six months ago when she began losing weight and finding it impossible to stop "peeing." Treated initially at the Coomb Hospital for bladder infections, she was eventually referred to Jervis Street and Mr. Walsh. "Finally," she said, "the ejiits found out what was wrong with me."

The warning: "Don't think of laying a finger on me until ya get a nurse down here," preceded the physical exam. The results appeared, in this student's estimation, normal, except for some weight loss.

An easy rapport developed between us in the days before her surgery. She wanted to know all about America. Tell me about the Grand Canyon and the Indians, she would ask, and does the desert really bloom? And have you heard the black people play jazz in New Orleans, and what about New York with its Broadway and the theater there? "Don't laugh at me, Yank," she said, "but I love the theater. I sneak into the Gaiety all the time. Siobhan McKenna's just smashing."

What I didn't know, I made up. Each day she sat Indian-style on the bed with a pillow pulled to her chest, in rapt attention. Her deep-set eyes, wide and focused, seemed totally immersed in the stories - like a sponge absorbing water.

One day I found her crying.

"What's wrong, Nora?"

"I'm going to die, Yank, I just know it."

"Oh stop it, Nora; Mr. Walsh is a fine surgeon."

She leaned forward, hunched over her knees.

"Who gives a damn anyway?" she asked. "Me dad's still ain't been to see me and my ma's just pissed I'm not around to take care of the feckin' kids." After a pause she looked up, "You sure I'll be alright, Yank?"

"Guaranteed."

A smile spread slowly across her face. "I'm too feckin' beautiful to die, ain't that right, Yank?"

"Absolutely, Nora."

Using the corner of the sheet, she dabbed her eyes. "Well, I guess that settles that."

With her surgery scheduled for the following morning, Nora asked if I would drop by that evening to wish her luck.

"Of course," I replied.

Dimmed lights scarcely outlined the beds as I quietly made my way down the ward. Since the census was low, unused beds and mattresses were stacked at intervals. Considerable distance separated the patients. Cool night air swayed the curtains of half-opened windows.

Nora turned quickly when I touched her shoulder. "Jasus," she said, "is that ya, Yank?"

"Shh... yes."

"What'n hell are you doing here in the middle of the night?"

"It's not that late," I answered. "Just be quiet." I pulled the curtains around and sat on the bed.

"Ya mad," she said. "If they catch you here, your arse is out of school and me-out of the hospital."

"Everything's taken care of Nora; brought the nurse a couple of Baby Chams. We'll be fine."

Moving to the head of the bed I put an arm around her shoulders and gave her cheek a quick peck. "Good to see you."

Snores were the only sounds in the half empty ward except for grunting and gasping noises from the bed across the way.

"What's wrong with that one?" I asked.

"Don't know," whispered Nora. "She was fine at tea and this began a bit ago... But," she continued, "it's me I'm feckin' worried about. They'll think I put ya up to this and who knows what they'll do."

"Look, I'll only be a couple of minutes, Nora. And listen, I brought you something." I retrieved a small bottle from inside my shirt and unscrewed the cap.

"What is it?" she asked.

"Just a little tonic." After a swallow I offered her the bottle. "It helps when you're nervous." She pushed my hand away.

"Nervous," she hissed, "I was asleep, ya ejiit."

Nora leaned toward me, "And don't you think ya're cute? Half jarred, with a little bottle handy, ready to slip into me bed."

"Only came to wish you luck. Like you asked." My hand slipped down her back, beneath the nightgown.

"But I didn't mean like that." Her voice seemed softer. "But," she continued, "I'm frightened for that lady over there."

Between the woman's gasps there now sounded an occasional gurgle.

"Ya got to do something, Yank."

"Do something? I'm not even supposed to be here." My hand dropped farther down her back.

"Well at least get the nurse!" She jerked my hand away.

I pulled back the curtains. The nurse's station was lit but empty. Across the way the woman was trying to push herself up in the bed, her face swollen and contorted in the effort.

As I approached she raised her arms and tried to speak; no sound emerged, only gasps; a white froth coated her lips. *Holy shit, she's drowning,* I realized.

Grabbing her beneath the shoulders I hauled her to the top of the bed, leaned her forward and shoved a pillow behind her back. After straightening the I.V. set-up that had pulled over, I found the clamp, jammed it shut, and ran to the nurse's station.

The nurse was in the kitchen having a cigarette.

"There's a woman feckin' dying out there!"

"Oh, good Jesus."

We ran back to the bed. "What happened?" she asked.

"How'n the hell do I know? I just arrived."

"I'll get the on-call and you, you get your bollocks out of here."

Nora was standing by the bed, hanging onto the curtain, as I ran by.

"Good luck in the morning, Nora."

The surgery went well. Mr. Walsh felt that the remaining kidney was free of disease. Post-operatively, the first three days were a blur of pain, dry heaves and headache. "Just leave me alone," she pleaded. The fourth day brought the change: color returned, pain eased, and the nurse said, "You wouldn't believe what she had for breakfast."

Mr. Walsh was very pleased with himself that day. "Nora," he said, "you look like a new woman." After he poked around her belly, he turned to the group and announced his surgical accomplishment. "Gentlemen, we have a good result," he said. "And I have to add, our Nora is something of a hero, you know. The night before her surgery, it seems a poor soul took a turn for the worse. Our little Nora heard her distress, pulled her up in bed, and went for help." He turned to Nora and said, "You did a fine job."

"Yes sir."

"But what amazed me is the strength it took," Knocky continued. "I was told the woman was all of twelve stone (168 pounds)." He patted her head. "But God does give us strength in times of crisis, does He not, Nora?"

She smiled. "Yes, sir. He does work in mysterious ways sometimes."

Nora's bag was packed, ready for discharge. And she looked wonderful: cheeks filled out, eyes bright, no darkness beneath them, hair tied in a pony tail.

"You should be hospitalized more often," I said. "You look terrific."

"So, d'ya want to see me again, Yank?"

"I would."

"I'll keep it in mind," she said, smiling. Then the nurse came to help her with her bag and Nora was gone.

The fourth medical year, the winter session of which commenced in October, included academics (Pediatrics, Psychiatry, Public Health: Social Preventive and Forensic Medicine, Obstetrics/Gynecology, Medicine, and Surgery), along with concomitant clinical exposure. The summer session - March to June - comprised clinical instruction in ophthalmology and aural surgery at the Eye and Ear Hospital and a course in pediatrics in a children's hospital.

I decided to defer the June Public Health exam to a later date and concentrate on the Pharmacology re-take, necessitated by the amphetamine-fueled disaster of the previous year. (Tom and I were successful on the repeat, and in something of a face-saving redemption I managed to cop Honors.)

In the Dublin universities during the 1960s and before, there existed a category of student, who in the parlance of the day, were designated "chronics." A relatively small cohort, they attended school for a protracted period without particular concern as to when they might graduate. Years ago there wasn't a time requirement for academic progression and graduation. If tuition was maintained, so too was one's status as a student. As a result of accreditation criteria and increasing applications, this unique group has passed into student lore. Although they existed in all academic areas of Dublin's colleges, it was specifically the chronic medical student at the Royal College of Surgeons with whom this writer was most familiar.

The chronic student could be placed in either of two categories. Both were defined by an extended academic chronology but one group included a more complex component. Students, who by reason of bad luck and indifferent study, had fallen behind a year or two, could not be considered a bona fide chronic on that basis alone. They, in most instances, were still striving and as was often noted, once the anatomy and physiology portion of the curriculum had been passed, had little difficulty with the ensuing clinical years.

The true chronic, on the other hand, transcended the usual urgency of exam success; passing, once an imperative, had become an option. They chose an alternative path, one less tedious and burdensome, more refined and leisurely, and better suited to their temperament. They would qualify when the time was right and wouldn't be rushed in the process.

If one word could be used to describe these gentlemen students, "relaxed" would be apt. Mornings they were readily identified enjoying rounds of coffee in the cafeteria, followed by lengthy sessions of snooker in the common room, or perhaps stretched out on a couch intently studying the daily racing line. Occasionally they were detected at clinical rounds in one of the hospitals. Clean-shaven, appropriately dressed, with a stethoscope peeking from their jacket or a tongue depressor protruding from a shirt pocket, they had the look and accessories of qualification already in place.

Theirs was a wide-ranging anecdotal knowledge in all areas of medical curricula, which they readily dispensed. They had the "book," to use a gambling term, on the examination tendencies of the professors: the areas from which examination questions were historically derived and the "tricks" meant to confuse, employed during the orals.

"They show you x-rays of the belly - either obstruction or ileus. Only ones the ejiits can read. But watch out for old Pringle (the surgery professor), sometimes, on the sly, he'll turn one around before he starts his questions. Look for the stomach air – that's the key. Chest x-ray seems scattered with bubbles? Probably bronchiectasis. Any heart murmur: act perplexed but always say diastolic. They wouldn't have asked if it were anything else. You're asked for an origin? Young patient, go with mitral valve, older person - aortic's always a good bet."

These insights were dispensed with the confidence and certainty of a bettor with inside information, placing ten quid on a horse at Leopardstown. If their tip went to ground, it would be excused as would a muddy track. The next time, the examiner, like the horse, would revert to form.

The chronic, by virtue of longevity, achieved a certain celebrity. Years in the trenches, they had suffered the slings and arrows, but in their fashion had continued to fight the good fight. They viewed their careers not in a negative way, but as having positive value. In conversation, one sensed a patronizing superiority, and paradoxically, an intimation that the breadth of their experience provided a clinical facility lacking in those who took the less circuitous route.

Admiration would be too strong a sentiment to attach to this group of ne'er-do-wells, but a measure of respect and perhaps a twinge of jealousy was, at least in my case, a reasonable tribute. Defying convention, accomplishing things - or not - on your own terms, and flaunting individuality are commendable traits. It's a luxury few students can avail themselves of, but for those who can - God bless 'em.

The ability to maintain a protracted medical education required creativity, resourcefulness and a certain panache. Tales of bad luck, unrealistic examinations and vindictive professors eventually wore thin for even the most beneficent of benefactors. A common ploy was to intermittently inform parents of examination success, whether real or imagined. The mix of a couple of failed exams with the occasional successful one was good for an additional three or four years. This was especially attractive for the foreign student whose home was thousands of miles away. However, for those from Ireland and the British Isles, it required considerable dexterity.

Some chronics achieved legendary status. One classic tale involved a student from Australia, who after some years, was bereft of further stratagems to placate his increasingly impatient parents. In desperation, he informed them that he had finally graduated, with Honors no less, and had established a practice in Dublin. The start-up costs for the practice were considerable, and funding, he told them, might become necessary for an indeterminate period. His plan, in real life, was to qualify through Apothecary's Hall (the reputably less rigorous, licensing body) in a year or two, and start a practice in Dublin. He assumed no one would be the wiser.

When his parents heard the news they were both relieved and delighted. Immediately, plans were made to visit him and his new practice. Not wanting to disappoint them, the new "Doctor," in cahoots with an established physician in Dublin, made arrangements to spend time in that office while his parents were in town. The ruse, it was said, worked to perfection. Whether or not the parents continued to contribute to his nascent medical career, I never learned.

The day of the chronic has long past. This group that lent counterpoint and leavened a fairly rigid medical curriculum has been reduced to anecdote and the reminiscence of a more relaxed time. But somehow one feels no sad songs need be sung. Physicians or not, it's six to four they're still enjoying the good life with fond memories of the grand time they had in Dublin, the adventure of their years at the College of Surgeons, and what might have been - if only they had more time.

Some weeks later, returning to my room, I found a note slipped under the door, from the hospital porter. A message had been received, it read, requesting I call the attached phone number. The following day I dialed the number; there was no mistaking the voice at the other end. "It's yer patient," she began. "D'ya remember me?"

"Of course, Nora. How've you been?" A chat ensued during which we arranged to meet the following Friday night at a pub in her neighborhood.

The Public House was in Dolphin's Barn, a working-class neighborhood in Dublin. When I arrived she was sitting at the far end of the bar, her face reflected in the mirror opposite, a yellow dress hung loosely.

"Thanks for coming, Yank."

"Good to see you, Nora." The kiss on her cheek brought a hint of perfume.

The air was thick with smoke as we pushed through the crowd to the lounge. Nora said she would claim the table being cleared by the back wall while I got the drinks.

Once settled, I raised my glass. "To Knocky," I toasted.

"Wouldn't he be surprised now if he saw the two of us here?" she asked with a smile.

"He would," I replied. "And not a little bit jealous of his student, I might add."

When I asked about the surgery she said things were going well but she had no energy. "Between the job and the kids, I'm destroyed."

It was true; across the table was not the Nora of four weeks earlier. Gone was the full face and the bright, sparkling eyes. Red lipstick only heightened her paleness and I noticed a tremor when she lit her cigarette.

"And ya," she asked, "with the exciting life?"

"Not so exciting: an exam in a couple weeks, then the Rotunda for obstetrics."

"Ah, but the time's going by and soon you're away."

She sipped her stout, licking the foam from her upper lip. "Reminds me of a play I saw at the Gate. From the Blaskets the man was. God forsaken rocks they are, off the west coast. Then one day, to America he went, his new bride left behind, believing his promise to return. Months, then years, she waited and prayed and walked the shore, crying for a man she hardly knew, waiting for a ship that never returned." Nora lit a cigarette. "Sad story, ain't it, Yank? I cried at the end." Nora shook her head, looked at me and smiled. "And it's to the grand life ya'll be going, and leaving no brides behind."

The lounge was packed with men in from work, bent over their pints at the small tables. An occasional shout or burst of laughter punctuated the hum of their conversations. Nora gestured toward them with her cigarette. "And this will be my lot."

"You'll do fine, Nora. You're a beautiful woman."

"Bullshit Yank; I'll end up with one of these charmers: boyos with money for porter and nothing else, and me in some tenement, schemin' supper for his Highness when he decides to stumble in. And then, of course, ready to spread me legs when he thinks he's feck'n Errol Flynn at two o'clock in the morning. Depressin' altogether it is."

After a moment she reached over and took my hand. "Pay no attention to me, Yank. Didn't I meet ya now; didn't ya make me laugh; and didn't ya open the window a little to let me see beyond the dirty old Liffey - even though your intentions weren't that feckin' upstanding?"

"You may get to some of those places we talked about. It's a twisting road we travel. You never know."

"Yank," she declared, "it'll only happen in me dreams."

Halfway through the second pint Nora got quiet.

"Anything wrong?" I asked.

"No," she replied, "but I have something I want to ask ya."

Leaning forward she spoke quickly. "You'll be missing your American Thanksgiving. I want ya to have it at my house, with me family."

"No need, Nora," I answered. "I'll have a few bob and we can go out some place."

This was dismissed with a shake of her head. "I want to show off the Yank I've talked so much about. Pa will be there and some people from the tenement downstairs. They've all heard about ya. Won't be fancy but ma will bring fresh stuff off the cart, and God help me, I'll try and cook a feckin' bird." She paused, her dark eyes intense. "It'll mean an awful lot to me."

"I've got exams."

"What's a few hours for Jasus sake."

I took one of her Woodbines and lit it. "Nora, we've got a date."

We walked to the top of her street, a long line of tenement houses with shops beneath, an occasional patch of green in front. In the distance poked the smoke stack of the Jacobs Biscuit Factory. Balancing on her toes she gave me a kiss on the cheek. "Goodbye, Yank, 'til Thanksgiving." She started to walk away then stopped and looked back. "Ya promise me?" she asked. I nodded. She shook her head "no." "The words," she insisted, "I need to hear the words."

I took a step toward her. "It's a promise."

She turned away. I watched as the yellow dress faded into the gray evening.

The call from the American Embassy was unexpected. The Ambassador was hosting a Thanksgiving dinner at the Gresham Hotel and invitations would be forthcoming to those Americans interested in joining him. The lady phoning informed me there would be an open bar, a turkey dinner with all the trimmings and a band for dancing. Also in attendance would be a group of Aer Lingus stewardesses. Without a moment's hesitation, I accepted.

A two-month clerkship in an obstetric hospital was required before being allowed to sit the Obstetrics/Gynecology exam. The three major maternity hospitals in Dublin at the time were the Rotunda, Hollis Street, and the Coomb. The Rotunda, established in the late 1700s, was the first maternity hospital in the United Kingdom, and at one time, the largest and most prestigious in Europe. Located at the north end of Dublin's O'Connell Street, it comprised two buildings: the hospital proper and an adjacent domed structure from which the hospital derived its name. Originally used as an entertainment and social center for hospital fund-raising activities, the facility, through various incarnations, evolved into the Gate Theater, a venue for some of Ireland's greatest playwrights. A.J. Cronin and W. Somerset Maugham, both physicians in their younger days, were two of the Rotunda's more distinguished alumni. With such a reputation and illustrious pedigree it became for me, as for many other Surgeons students, an easy choice.

In contrast to medicine and surgery where an easy familiarity had developed over the clinical years, ob-gyn was a relative unknown. Whatever knowledge the student might possess was gained primarily through anecdote or hearsay, usually presented as an obstetric catastrophe or raunchy sexual aberration.

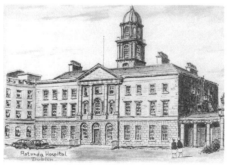

Rotunda Hospital - Dublin

Students were required to deliver ten babies, supervised by a midwife, which when accomplished, allowed participation in deliveries outside the hospital, "in the district." After attendance at a series of lectures and births, my time arrived, and along with two others, I retired to a small room near the delivery area, to wait until summoned. Excepting meals and physical necessities, we remained in the room until we completed the prescribed number. Such was the fecundity of Irish women, the requirement was usually satisfied within two or three days.

Midwives ruled the delivery room. Their reputation and our ignorance no doubt heightened the effect; but their physical presence - large women, thick forearms, spade-like hands, imperious manner, voices that resonated with authority - certainly fostered intimidation.

Inconspicuously, I eased to the back of the delivery room.

"Och, a new one." The voice originated from a massive figure garbed in white. Two others in the room turned to look at me. "First time, Mister?"

Not wishing to chance a stutter, I nodded.

"Well, Mister," she boomed, "get yourself ready and be quick about it. Our little mother won't be waiting long."

Deliveries in Dublin hospitals at that time were accomplished with mothers lying on their left sides, the left lateral position. Aside from some physiological and anatomic advantages, it allowed for a more controlled delivery and lessened the possibility of a perineal tear. This was a special advantage when deliveries took place in the home, for if a tear occurred, the on-call registrar at the hospital had to be called out for the repair. Those requests were never received kindly.

Gloved and gowned I waited, hands clasped as if in prayer, while Bridget, the midwife in charge, who allowed that familiarity, hovered over, examined, and cajoled the mother-to-be. Another white-garbed woman was present who introduced herself as Mary.

Finally, Bridget turned to me. "Mister, I think we're ready." Directing me to the end of the table, she nodded toward a circle of emerging scalp; then she motioned for me to stand behind the woman, now lying on her side. Draping my left arm over her swollen belly, she placed my right hand on the woman's lower back.

"Do you feel it?" Bridget asked.

"Feel what?" I replied.

"The chin."

I shook my head.

Bridget took my thumb and placed it against something I did not recognize.

"The chin?" I asked.

"Yes, Mister, the chin." She muttered something under her breath.

At Bridget's direction I pushed on this newly discovered piece of anatomy while applying pressure with my left hand. The infant's head began to emerge. The perineum stretched and soon was paper-thin; some fibers began to separate in the mid-line.

"No more pushing," Bridget commanded the mother. Then she moved my hand onto the crown of the head. "Now Mister," she said, "keep good pressure and let's ease it out slow."

My right hand, I became aware, wasn't near anything that remotely resembled a chin, the thumb numb, unable to bend. Pressure was maintained with the other, and with Bridget's hand over mine, the perineum slowly stretched over the infant's head and then there it was, delivered without a tear. Sweat was rolling down my forehead, burning my eyes. My other hand fell away from the woman's back. The thumb, pushed back, seemed locked in place.

"Now, Mister, what do you do?"

A specific sequence followed the delivery of the head. To start, hands were washed in a nearby basin, after which a bulb syringe was used to clean out the mouth. In my haste, the hand washing part was forgotten and I went straight for the syringe. Bridget intercepted my move in mid-course with a whopping thump.

Hands washed, the next step was pretty straight-forward. The bulb on the syringe, once compressed, is inserted into the infant's mouth, the pressure released and secretions are sucked up. I failed to do this. Not until the syringe tip was well inside the baby's mouth, did I squeeze the bulb. This scattered whatever secretions there were to God knows where.

"Mother of God," hissed Bridget in a half whisper, so the mother wouldn't hear. "D'ya want to kill the poor child altogether, you ejiit?" Grabbing the syringe she quickly sucked out whatever I had missed.

Mentally shaken, vision clouded, legs suspect, hand numb, mouth parched - "would I be able to finish" was one of my scattered thoughts.

The new mother quiet to this point, interrupted, "Do you know what I had yet?" Her voice seemed as parched as mine.

"Not yet, Mrs.," replied Bridget. "Take a deep breath and give me a little push; then we'll know." With that effort, which included a short cry of pain, the infant emerged, its debut announced by a high pitched squeal.

"It's a boy, you've got Mrs.," announced Bridget, "and a fine one it is." The grey-scummed, puffy-faced, heavy-lidded infant was lifted up for the mother to see.

"Thank God," she said smiling, "My third try - finally a boy. The old man would kill me if I brought home another girl."

"Hope he looks like him, Dearie," interjected Mary.

The patient, now rolled onto her back, laughed, "Me too."

"What's next, Mister?" asked Bridget, nodding toward a basin in which cotton balls were floating. These I knew were used to clean the baby's eyes immediately after delivery. Two of the cotton balls were secured, just before my wayward elbow struck the side of the basin. Water soon covered a sizeable portion of the floor. Bridget stared at me, seemed about to say something harsh, then shook her head and turned away.

After the cord was tied - double knotted with two ties on the baby's side - Bridget let me cut the cord. Using one hand to steady the other, this was accomplished without incident.

Gingerly, I picked up the infant and handed him to a nurse who wrapped him in a blanket and brought him to his mother for a short visit before taking him to the nursery.

"Still not finished," Bridget informed me. Directing me to place my left hand over the uterus she placed the umbilical cord in the other. "Massage," she said, "and pull gently."

In short order, the cord lengthened and the afterbirth followed, spread like a giant red jellyfish in the waiting basin.

"Keep massaging," Bridget decreed and walked away.

My legs, like strands of licorice, offered little support. The patient's eyes were closed, apparently sleeping. I leaned over her for support as I worked on the uterus with the heel of each hand. She opened her eyes.

"Sorry." I said, straightening up.

"You're fine," she said. "You helped deliver my baby didn't you?"

"A little - I'm a student but they let me assist some," I answered, thinking *if you only knew*. "And now," I said, feigning brightness, "you have a handsome little man."

"Thanks to..." she moved her gaze around the room, with a nod to those in attendance... "and even you," she hesitated, "my young doctor to be."

Embarrassed, I looked up quickly but no one was within earshot.

Finally Bridget came over, felt the uterus, and said I could stop the massage.

Then the fourth stage of labor, as it was popularly called, washing down, in a large sink, the red rubber sheet which had been placed under the mother during the delivery.

Bridget approached and placed a hand on my shoulder. "Okay, Mister, you got through your first."

I nodded. *My God*, I thought, *I'll never survive another.* "Bridget," I asked, my voice raspy, "d'ya think the baby will be alright, you know, me pushing all that stuff into his lungs?"

"He'll be fine." For an instant I sensed a smile behind her mask. "And by the way, Mister, you did alright. The first one's always the toughest." She removed her mask and she *was* smiling. "Hope we can work together again sometime."

After changing my clothes, I made my way to the room where the others were waiting, stopping outside the door for a moment to steady myself.

"How'd it go?" asked one.

Collapsing into a chair I reached for the cigarettes in my jacket.

"Any problems?" asked the other.

Looking up at their earnest faces I allowed a small smile. "Nothing to it," I replied, "feckin' piece of cake."

Over the next two days, without drama or mishap, the required deliveries were accomplished. Although exhausted at the end, it was a good tired. All the midwives said I'd done well, and though perhaps the standard line, I agreed with them - the first sense of accomplishment in my fledging medical career.

With the in-house ten-delivery requirement accomplished, we were allowed to participate in deliveries in Dublin's inner city: the "district." District calls were categorized as either normal or abnormal. A call to the hospital which indicated the possibility of a complication, usually bleeding, would fall into the abnormal category and was handled by the obstetric registrar (resident) accompanied by a nurse and a student. The normal category consisted of ladies with an uneventful pre-natal course who had gone into labor. Two students accompanied by a nurse, usually a midwife in training, attended the delivery in the patient's home. Having been followed at the Rotunda pre-natally, the record of those visits and their obstetric history was available. In almost every instance these ladies had prior uncomplicated deliveries: thus, it was assumed this birth would be a straight-forward event with no surprises. Students rotated through a schedule; when your name came up you remained in the hospital or in close proximity. The on-call wait was often accomplished at Mooney's, a pub across the street from the Rotunda. Arrangements were made with the hospital porter to come get you when the call came through.

The deliveries, in most cases, occurred in Dublin's poorest sections. It was not unusual for a family of four, five, or more, to be crowded into a two-room dwelling with shared toilet facilities and no electricity. In addition to our portable delivery kit, we always brought along a large battery-powered lamp.

On arrival, the nurse immediately assessed the degree of cervical dilatation and the imminence of delivery via a rectal exam. The students, in their turn, repeated the examination. Sheets of newspapers were spread on the bed beneath the mother. The lamp was placed on a chair or table at the end of the bed, its light focused on the delivery area. The only medications given were a quarter grain of morphine and atropine.

As news of the impending delivery made its way through the tenements, neighbors soon converged in the home, usually the kitchen. Children could often be heard as they played in the hallway, while a doorless room allowed quick peeks and accompanying giggles.

The nurse supervised the students as they shared the delivery, exchanging roles as events proceeded. In most instances, it was a full hands-on experience for the student. The nurse only intervened to demonstrate technique or to offer advice. The post-delivery care for the new-born was provided by the nurse.

Once it was ensured that the baby was fine and the mother stable with a hard uterus, we joined the group in the kitchen for a cup of tea. The polite, "And would you like something with it?" was usually accompanied by bread or biscuits. Then back to the hospital. Later, we might enjoy a pint or two at Mooney's as we recounted our experience.

Students followed the particular baby they helped deliver over the next ten days, accompanying the pediatric nurse on her post-natal rounds, often another ten to twelve calls. This provided a great introduction to post-natal care, and of course, it was neat for students to follow the baby they helped bring into the world.

The Rotunda offered a great clinical program, but, beyond that, the exposure to Dublin's inner city and the abject circumstances in which much of that population lived, introduced me to an unfamiliar reality. Our deliveries were accomplished in tenements, uniform in their squalor: dark, dirty spaces which sweltered and stank in the summer, most without heat in the winter; walls, where pictures seldom hung, gashed and fissured; windows either broken or boarded. Furniture - a table and a chair or two - was concentrated in the kitchen; a single bed or mattresses strewn on the floor identified the sleeping area. And here was the lady of the house adding another kid to the two or three running barefoot around the place. What, in the name of God, you wondered, were they thinking? Of course, thinking had little to do with it. As Ireland was predominantly a Catholic country, birth control was not available. (Condoms made their legal appearance in 1970, obtainable only by prescription.)

Particular moments are indelible: the lady, bed-ridden for ten days prior to her delivery, hair undulating, thick with maggots; the roll, offered with tea, one end having been gnawed on by a frequently seen rodent. Thankfully, noticed also by the new father, the used portion was promptly cut away, re-served...and not half bad.

But it was marvelous training with full credit given to the midwives. They made the system work, as doctors alone could never have handled the obstetric volume of the city. At the completion of our residency, a certificate was presented. The party which followed was largely stocked with small bottles of Guiness taken from the wards, stout given as a dietary supplement to patients at the time.

Probably abetted by the OB experience, my new-found compatibility with the clinical side of medicine continued to germinate - not in full flower, by any stretch, but taking hold with a good chance of survival. The academics maintained their challenge but were quite doable with a modicum of effort on my part. So perhaps Aunt Bertha was right when she predicted that eventually my ambivalence regarding medicine as a career would resolve itself.

A Broth of a Boy

M iss Halligan had held my place in the digs while I was at the Rotunda. When I returned to my room, I found a large body stretched out on the second bed, snoring. I was soon to meet my new roommate, Max Mallory.

Max was from the seacoast town of Wexford. He claimed to be descended from the Vikings, who in the 700s A.D., raped, burned, and pillaged their way along Ireland's east coast. And with his blonde hair, fair complexion, ruddy cheeks, and watery-blue eyes, there was a resemblance. Max, a medical student, had been in pursuit of his degree for the past five years.

His academic career had begun at University College Dublin, and prior to his final year, for reasons never divulged, he dropped out and continued his studies at Apothecary's Hall. The examining body mentioned earlier, conducted exams in medicine, surgery, and obstetrics and then permitted successful candidates to dispense drugs in a chemist shop and practice medicine in England and Ireland.

Max stayed with Miss Halligan whenever he returned to prepare for examinations. Two interests, she maintained, impeded his academic progress: a fondness for the brew and playing the horses. On each visit, expectations were high. Miss Halligan insisted that Max made commendable efforts, but just before the exam, inexplicably, he "took to the drink," skipped the exam, went home, only to return for another try some months later.

A "broth of a boy" was Max. His personality exhibited a mix of ingredients: a gift for repartee and story-telling, charm in the guise of back-handed compliments, sarcasm that passed for humor, a tentative self-esteem improved with alcohol, sporadic intelligence, bouts of moodiness, and healthy dollops of depression - arguably a well- balanced Irishman.

Max suffered hangovers, which although short-lived, were

for the ages. A typical morning scenario: Max stretched out on his bed, fully clothed and snoring. Eventually rousing himself, he'd attempt to stand, his body shaking as if chilled. Eyes scarcely visible in a puffy face, he'd find his way to the sink, fill it with cold water, into which he'd repeatedly and rapidly thrust his face. Hands on each faucet protected his head, his blonde hair would stretch over his forehead, and water would soak his shirt and pants. The closest re-enactment I've seen of his ritual was Paul Newman, in the movie, *The Sting*, resolving a hangover in similar fashion, except he used ice cubes.

Occasionally, this procedure was repeated two or three times. Finally his lips would move. "Jasus," he'd say, voice quivering, "I'm in a terrible way altogether." Then sitting on the side of the bed, head between his hands, Max would recount the adventures of the previous night and tell of the "shites up from the country," who had brought him to this sorry state.

When color returned to his cheeks and his eyes allowed light, he'd think of nourishment. "Sure, I know," he'd say, "I've missed Miss Halligan's elegant breakfast but maybe she'd give us a bit of tea. A cut or two of the soda bread would be grand right now. Let's go down and say good morning to Kitty." And of course, she would fix him some breakfast.

Max had a way with the ladies, the charm of the rogue. Lorna, a middle-aged spinster, was another of our long term residents who worked as a clerk in Dublin. Visions of marriage persisted but, she admitted, chances were diminishing. Lorna maintained her appearance, always well-groomed, with perhaps a year or two left before abandoning the tight skirts she favored.

"Ah, Lorna, you're looking grand tonight," exclaimed Max when she arrived for tea. "Jasus, you're a fine figure of a woman."

"Oh, go away out of that, Max," she'd reply. But you could see the half smile and we knew she was loving it.

"How the lads in Louth let a fine thing like you escape?" Max shook his head in mock disbelief. "Dumb bog men altogether." And on he would go, all in good fun with no offense taken.

When Max was my roommate during this stay at Hyde House, he was preparing for an obstetrics exam. No distractions this time around, he resolved. Max *did* make a commendable effort: most nights he studied in the UCD library and attended rounds and clinics during the day. Lecture notes were kept in a 6" by 8" spiral notebook along with addresses, women's phone numbers, horse's names, and notations of bets placed. Occasionally I saw Max at Hollis Street, an Obstetric Hospital, when teaching rounds were in progress. Standing at the periphery, notebook in hand (into which he occasionally scribbled), he appeared quite absorbed in the proceedings. The same absorption was similarly noted when seen chatting up the nurses, also with note-book in hand.

One of the nurses at the time was from the Wexford area. She, according to Max, had visions of their returning to establish a practice there. The nurse, it so happened, had an aunt who was a char lady (cleaning lady) in the employ of Mr. De Valera, who was not only the son of Eamon DeVelera, Prime Minister of Ireland at the time, but also an examiner in obstetrics at various medical schools in Dublin, including " Pots" Hall. Once aware of this, Max persuaded the woman to be on the lookout in her cleaning duties for any papers that might relate to examinations. Coincidentally, at the time, the char lady was having an altercation with the good doctor over wages.

Some weeks later I was awakened by Max shaking my bed. "I've got it!" His voice was a hushed scream. "By the sweet Jasus, I've got it."

"Got what?" I asked, squinting in the light.

"The feckin' exam is what. Oh, sweet mother!" He handed me a single piece of paper.

Under the heading, Obstetrics and Gynecology Examination, Apothecary's Hall, with a date approximately two weeks hence, were a series of neatly typed questions. "I'll be damned," is all I could say.

For obvious reasons, Max decided against advertising the fact that he had the exam. Selling the questions to a select few was considered but rejected with a firm, "I'm taking no chances on a leak." He also decided to stop studying.

I was away at the time the examination was given. On my return, Max's things were not in the room. Miss Halligan was in the kitchen preparing tea.

"Max...," I started.

"Before you ask," her voice exasperated, "he didn't take the exam."

I was incredulous. "But, why not?"

The night before the exam, she recounted, Max had a few drinks with a man who exercised horses for Vincent O'Brien, the legendary Irish horse trainer. The man gave Max a tip "as solid as sterling" on a two-year-old racing the following day at the Curragh. "Dead cert," Max was told. "So off our boyo goes."

"Why didn't he go to Kilmartins (a licensed betting establishment) down the street?"

"Who knows? That's Max. Anyway, he pawned everything he owned. Even borrowed a few quid from me and off to the Curragh."

"So did the horse win?"

Miss Halligan shook her head. "No. Max said something about the regular jockey not being available and the replacement was inexperienced and couldn't handle the horse."

"Just unbelievable. So where's he now?"

"He didn't say, but other times he's usually gone to England."

(I never saw Max again. On a visit to Ireland a few years later, I asked Miss Halligan about him. She said he had stopped by and told her that he'd given up medicine and was moving to Canada.)

During the fourth year, I joined our class rugby team as did Pat O'Brien and a couple of other hearty souls. Being a fast runner I was placed out on the wing; far removed from the muck and maul of the scrum, where large, strong people attempted to wrest control of a pumpkin-sized, bloated ball. The side achieving possession makes a series of lateral passes to a line of runners who attempt to move the ball past the goal line, resulting in a score or "try." The last person on this line was me. Personal protective equipment was non-existent.

Rugby was, and remains, a very popular sport with intense international competition between countries such as England, Scotland, Wales, Australia, and South Africa. The star of Ireland's national team at that time was Tony O'Reilly who also played out on the wing: no fool, he!!

A RUGBY TALE

The Purefoy Cup was an intra-mural competition, the winner of which was designated the best rugby team in the college. My memory of the year I was a member of the team that won the Cup has scarcely diminished; rather it's been enhanced, as is often the case when one becomes older.

A bright sun shone that day on the sward of green pitch, the centerpiece of Surgeon's athletic complex at Byrd Avenue in Clonskeagh. An enthusiastic crowd was in attendance, their anticipation palpable. Finally, 1:00 p.m – a crescendo of cheers shook the stands, and the match began.

Fiercely fighting, the scrums dominated the action: wheeling about, advancing and retreating, with the occasional break-out stymied before it extended to the players on the wing. Increasingly restive, with but a few minutes left to play, the crowd implored their favored team to score, as neither had. Finally, the moment never forgotten: the break-out started with a quick feed from the scrum half; the ball, slathered with mud, passed one to the other along the wing - the final lateral and the ball was mine.

Clutching it to my side, I ran as never before. In spite of my effort, the horde pounded in hot pursuit, close enough that an occasional hand grazed my back. Mind and body, every synaptic connection, was focused on one thought: *out run the bastards and bring the trophy home.* But could I hold out?

My legs, as in a dream, felt bound in molasses. With the goal in sight I dug deep, found the strength reserved for such moments, and in a final burst of speed blazed over the white line for the try.

My teammates leaped on me, immersing me in gratitude. Modest in victory, I disdained their congratulations; a circumspect wave acknowledged the frenzied cheers of the multitude. The chap from the newspaper insisted on a photo for the morning paper.

Nice Try

The preceding rugby tale was just that, a tale, containing not a shred of truth. Rather, it is a Walter Mittey-esque depiction of the imagined athletic talents I brought to the rugby field. In various social settings over the years, the game has been re-enacted - with details occasionally enhanced. Time and distance, I reasoned, would diminish the possibility of a challenge.

The facts, more mundane, had us playing on a gray, battle-scarred patch of pitch, the day beset by rain showers, attended by a "crowd" of perhaps twenty people. When, unfortunately, the ball came into my possession, I ran as fast as my skinny legs would allow, my mind totally focused on avoiding structural damage. Feigning injury and falling was given serious consideration. All concerns were eliminated when, by the grace of God, the goal line appeared, over which I managed to stumble. Even the try I made was tainted. After I scored and began to lope off the field I was suddenly tackled by a teammate, John Dillon.

"What the hell's wrong with you?" I shouted.

John, a great athlete, but a man of few words, just shook his head and walked away. Apparently, for a try to be official, the ball must be touched to the ground which I had failed to do. John's tackle brought contact with the ground both to the ball and me. So the congratulations I so richly deserved were heaped on John, for his quick thinking.

(At our recent 2011 reunion I dined with John and was tempted to recall the incident with him. After consideration I demurred. This is one of the few athletic events, with any factual basis, that I have left to embellish; why dredge up issues that might tarnish a perfectly fine fantasy, which over the years has become increasingly credible? The Purfoyle Cup medal I received, still in my possession, now serves as a pendent for a necklace worn by my wife on occasion.)

A n annual stage show was a college-sponsored event, meant to highlight the talents of various members of the student population. Many performances had a serious bent, such as light operatic offerings and Ian Henry's classical piano selections. Any quality the evening's program could boast started to erode when Cormac "Mooch" Brady gave his (actually excellent) interpretation of Billy Daniel's classic, "That Old Black Magic." I played the ukulele somewhat, and as part of a trio, offered show-stoppers such as "Tom Dooley" and "Five Foot Two."

The occasional skit was offered. One year a couple of us composed a mildly offensive piece in which three male cadavers, one night in the anatomy room, attempt to have their way with a newly arrived female cadaver, (classmate Nuala Kilcoyne) who had a body to die for. Since these Lothario's never knew what appendage might be detached the following day, their solicitations, by necessity, were more urgent than ardent. Their overtures, in any case, made little impression as Nuala, heartless to the end, dismissed the lot of them with the final words of the sketch. "Lads," she said, "you're a cool lot, and I appreciate the attention, but after you've seen one stiff you've seen them all." Such was the level of sophistication we brought to the assemblage.

Probably the most embarrassing episode occurred one year when Gary O'Connor, a year ahead of us and whose father Matthew O'Connor was the pathology professor, planned a rendition of Faustus's passionate soliloquy before his descent into Hell. Gary asked Pat and me to assist by representing two of Satan's acolytes, sent to seize Faustus and escort him to his fiery destination. Garbed in snug red tights we made our entrance. Almost immediately a problem became apparent. Pat was 6'4,

and I, 6'1; the tights were of medium size. Crouched in a men-
acing pose with arms raised, we advanced toward Faustus. Each
step we took resulted in the increased exposure of our buttocks,
in spite of frantic attempts to maintain modesty. This provoked
huge outcries and laughs from the audience, which rendered silent Gary's impassioned rendition. This did not sit well with Mr.
O'Connor, our apologies falling on deaf ears.

(At a recent Surgeons reunion I learned that Gary became a
psychiatrist, moved to the United States, did advanced work at
Johns Hopkins Hospital in Maryland, and fashioned a marvelous career in that specialty. Recently, he was named CEO and
Medical Director at the Betty Ford Clinic in Rancho Mirage,
California - a long way from the bright lights of the Surgeons'
stage and his Faustian misadventure.)

THE VICAR AND HIS DISCIPLE

During my last year of residence in Hyde House, an Anglican minister and his son stayed with us for approximately six months. The vicar, Miss Halligan informed us, was seventy-one and his son, Edward, somewhere in his 30's. The semblance was that of a grandfather and grandson. They kept to themselves and seldom joined us in the sitting room before tea but went directly to their table. As they waited for their tea, the vicar read from a black breviary while Edward jotted notes in a small book. Edward occasionally read the notes back to his father who listened with eyes closed and arms folded across a rotund mid-section.

Their dress was formal: the vicar in a dark suit with a white clerical collar and Edward in a pale gray suit with shirt and tie. A gold watch chain was suspended across both their vests. The vicar's squat frame was supported by tiny feet, usually in slippers. His unlined, pudgy face bore a fixed serene expression presumably reflecting an inner tranquility. Edward was tall, slightly bent with slick blond hair combed straight back over his scalp. His face was pale with patches of stubble, as if he hadn't used a mirror when he shaved. An occasional smile was tentative, barely exposing even white teeth. The perception was of youthful good looks caught up in the trappings of an older person.

Occasionally, Pat O'Brien, living at Hyde House at the time, and I would find Edward reading in the sitting room when we returned late in the evening from the library or the pub. His father had gone to bed and Edward, relaxed with a cigarette, would chat with us.

Although hesitant at first, he eventually shared his background. His father, he explained, had retired from a parish in County Monaghan and was waiting for an opening at a retirement home in England. Edward couldn't live with him there but would find lodging nearby. His mother had died of cancer when he was ten years of age. He described her as an outgoing, vivacious woman whose death extinguished any lightness or gaiety in the household. Since then, Edwards's life had been effectively cloistered and revolved completely around his father, who also provided his in-home education. Any social life he had, derived from church functions. Edward enjoyed an occasional cigarette, but he rarely drank alcohol and after being prodded, admitted he had never been alone with a woman.

The vicar's plan was to have Edward follow him into the ministry, but grades on entrance exams to various divinity schools were found to be wanting. More disquieting to his father, and for which Edward felt considerable guilt, was his lack of interest in the religious life. Efforts to foster his vocation, however, continued. The readings he transcribed in the evenings were meant for reflection and preparation for the call, which his father insisted would surely come. "I pray regularly and diligently," he said, "but nothing happens."

Socially removed, he was eager to know of the world outside as if curious of another culture. Pat and I, probably with considerable embellishment, told him of Dublin's night life: the pubs, the parties, and the eager women who filled the dance halls. He absorbed our stories, almost child-like in his naiveté.

Every so often, with his father's permission, he joined us on a night out, the purported destination being a movie or play. Rather, we took him to the pubs we frequented: Davy Byrnes or Frank Swift's Toby Jug. Edward would chat with Pat and me, but when others joined, he became quiet and withdrawn, speaking only if addressed. Almost foppish in his high-rise black shoes, suit, tie and gold chain, he sipped his pint and absorbed the scene.

Edward was aware of women. Often he fixed his stare so intently on a female it would cause her to giggle and whisper to her companion. He never initiated a conversation, just blended into the background. After one or perhaps two drinks he excused himself and left, never joining us for dances or parties; perhaps our invitations were half-hearted.

Edward enjoyed these occasions but there seemed a reticence, a perception that he wanted to experience the outside world but not too much. Perhaps he was fearful of getting caught up in a situation with which he couldn't cope, just as a long-term prisoner might feel when released into an unfamiliar world. After a few excursions with Pat and me, he never pushed to be included in further outings and seemed content to stay in his customary environment.

Fathers come in various packages, none tied with the same bow. Whatever's inside can't be returned for a new model. Observing the vicar, I thought he had ill-served his son, creating an anomaly totally unprepared for a world he would soon face alone. In retrospect, he was probably doing what he thought best - perhaps he knew no other way- so he shouldn't be faulted. And the obvious affection between the two - perhaps all that either needed or wanted - may well have been the legacy that sustained Edward in the years which followed. And so it is with most father-son relationships: by turns close and distant, emotionally awkward, replete with impatience, anger, and immaturity (equally shared) - but anchored with an unconditional love, that rarest of gifts. With that in place, the rest are but patches of fluky wind on a once-in-a-lifetime sail.

Eventually a vacancy opened in the Bath area of England and they left for their new residences. To the end, Edward was the dutiful son. Whether the few excursions into Dublin sparked any inclination for further adventures can only be conjecture. Probably not until his father died, we suspected. Being so pitifully equipped socially, his will certainly be a bumpy flight. Hopefully it ended well.

Farewell to Hyde House

Miss Halligan made the announcement at the end of tea one evening. "I've some bad news for all of you," she began. "Hyde House has been sold." She paused a moment, then continued, "And the new owner wants the place cleared out by the end of the month." It was now the middle of the month. "I was just notified a few days ago," she said, "and I've been looking for a place to move to, but so far there's nothing I can afford."

"So what's going to happen here?" someone asked. "Will it still be a digs?"

"I don't know the plans but it won't be a digs. Otherwise we wouldn't be asked to leave."

A few days later Miss Halligan returned to tell us she had found a place on South Circular Road. "Not as big, with fewer rooms," she said, "but the best I could do on short notice." She went on to say that the house had two large rooms on the second floor which could each accommodate three people and a living room on the first floor, suitable for another two. One of the two single rooms in the basement was hers; the other was to be occupied by her nephew Joe. A single bathroom was available on the second floor, a bathtub in the basement. "There will be no change in the rent," she concluded.

On hearing the news, the regulars, especially Frank and Lorna, were stunned. They had both been with Miss Halligan from the time they had moved to Dublin - over eight years ago in both instances. The unavailability of single rooms prompted them to seek other accommodations, which they fortunately found before the house closed. Dan Savage, also departing, was non-committal, but I believe he moved in with his girlfriend, whom he married within six months of his departure.

For my part, the decision was easy. I had decided some time

earlier to stay with Miss Halligan to the finish. She had been good to me and we enjoyed each other. Also, since things were going reasonably well academically, I didn't want to change my luck. Jim Orange also made the move with us.

A small party was held in the kitchen on the last night; we all chipped in for the stout and some wine for Lorna and Miss Halligan. Reminiscences were shared, with Frank Gillan being especially sentimental.

"Jasus," Frank said, "you've been good to us, Kitty, all these years." He seldom drank and was feeling it that night. "Do you remember..." and he went through a list of previous tenants, most of them females, whom he had enjoyed.

Dan, relentless to the end, couldn't resist a final skewer. "Maybe, Frank, you'll find yourself a little macusla (darling) in the new place. And get that hurley of yours (short for a hurling stick) working again."

Frank's face flushed; he seemed about to speak, then a broad grin spread across his craggy face. Going over to Dan, he gave him a hug. "Me oul'segosha (friend)," he said, "I'm going to miss you."

Dan put his arm around the big man's shoulder. "And I'll miss you too, you old bollocks."

Miss Halligan thanked those who were moving with her - a total of five. Until three more tenants were aboard she would, she said, have trouble making her own rent payments.

At the end of the evening we toasted Hyde House and all those who had darkened its doorstep over the years. Even Douglas Hyde himself had a glass raised in his honor. For me it was a grand place - my home for four years - where friends were made and good times had.

(Return trips to Dublin over the years have always included visits to the old haunts. Hyde House is now occupied by an insurance firm, its elegant Georgian facade besmirched with brown brick. The traditional windows conform to a contemporary office style, and strips of faux marble bound the wide front door. Thankfully the stained fan light remains with "Hyde House" retained over the transom. Despite the changes, little effort is required to recollect that bright September morning when a young man, standing on those very steps, asked a small, aproned woman if she had any room for him.)

I pushed a cart filled with my belongings past Harcourt Street and a gritty collection of shops. The walk to the new place was scarcely longer than twenty minutes, but a world apart from the tranquility of my former neighborhood. A major artery into the city, on the bus line, South Circular Road resounded with the screech and blare of traffic; the street was strewn with litter. Just beyond Synge Street, and the home where George Bernard Shaw was born, I reached my destination. A nondescript structure, it was one of a long line of attached residences that stretched half the block. Many had businesses advertised in their first floor windows. A large church loomed across the street.

I shared a room with Jim Orange and a recent arrival. The room, absent a sink, with one closet, and a couple of feet between beds, made for an intimate living situation. Bedbugs, in residence at the time of our arrival, were a recurring feature until they succumbed to a variety of sprays or more likely to the sinus-clearing stench of the socks and shoes of the new roommate. When apprised of our discomfort, he obliged and at bedtime put his shoes and the accompanying socks on the sill, then opened the window. Although his effort was appreciated it made little difference. Whether coincidental or not is uncertain, but my olfactory sense, previously acute, subsequently became less so.

All the transfers from Hyde House found the new place adequate, but all agreed, absent was the look, the feel, the "characters," and dare I say, the charm of the place on Adelaide Road.

My intent that summer, before starting the final year in the fall, was to find a clerk position in a hospital. On the recommendation of a female English student I met at the Rotunda, I applied to various hospitals, both in England and Wales. They were chronically in need of help, and in return, room and board were provided; some even offered a small stipend. In due course I received an acceptance from the Royal Albert Infirmary in Wigan, County Lancashire, on the west coast of England.

The Infirmary was a 75-bed hospital serving Wigan and the surrounding area. An attractive two-bedroom apartment, a short distance from the hospital, was assigned to me. A kitchenette was included, but if preferred, meals could be taken at the hospital cafeteria. The princely sum of three pounds a week was an additional bonus.

Two other Irish medical students, one from University College Cork; the other from University College Dublin, and a recently qualified English physician, Arthur Reynolds, welcomed me on my arrival. Each student was assigned to a physician with medical and surgical registrars available for assistance. As outlined by the senior registrar, our job as students was to perform histories and physicals on new admissions, arrange routine lab work, and present the patient to the physician on his rounds. In-patients under his care were seen daily; our note in the medical record verified the visit. An Emergency Room rotation was established, and with surgeon approval, we were allowed to assist at surgery.

I was assigned to a Dr. Dick with whom I worked for the major part of my time in Wigan. Affable in manner, competent by reputation, probably in his late fifties, he specialized in gastro-intestinal disorders, specifically stomach ulcers. Whether or not he was certified in that specialty I never determined, but this was the particular niche he had created for himself. Dr. Dick's treatment for virtually all gastro-intestinal problems was a milk drip: A Levine tube passed through the patient's nose to their stomach. Milk from a large open-mouthed container was then dripped, via the tube, into the stomach twenty-four hours a day, for days at a time. It was not unusual to see four or five patients in the ward with drips in progress. Since those days it has been pretty much established that milk increases acid secretions and probably is not the ideal treatment for gastric ulcers. Many patients, however, indicated relief from their symptoms. Then again, they may simply have been sick of milk and wanted to go home.

On the social side, I became friendly with one of the ward nurses: a tall, blonde, English girl. A relatively benign relationship ensued; her good looks a trophy to display at the random hospital party. As for male friends, Arthur Reynolds, the newly-minted English physician, loved his golf, and endowed with a vehicle, he and I flailed away at various local courses. On nights off, unfortunately influenced by the two Irishmen, we managed to improve the bottom line of a number of local pubs.

Also at the Royal Albert that summer was a Chinese woman, Jane (I don't recall her last name), who had graduated from Surgeons three years earlier; I remembered she was a student instructor in the physiology lab. She was now the medical registrar at the infirmary. A friendship developed to the extent of a movie or coffee in town. As much as the recollection pains me, when we were together in public, I was embarrassed to be with her - an Oriental. This was in the late 1950s and walking with someone who didn't match your skin color caused heads to turn along with the occasional comment - at least that was my perception. Being such a sensitive jerk, it bothered me, and I stopped seeing her socially.

Jane was a totally fine person: highly intelligent and a great teacher. Although not required, but at her insistence, I made rounds with her each day.

"Physiology is the bedrock of medicine," she insisted. "Disease is physiology with a problem." The car mechanic analogy: "You can't fix a car if you don't know how it works," was trotted out frequently. For example, if the patient had a renal problem, her first query would be: "How does a normal kidney work? Follow a drop of urine for me." With that established, the next question was: "So what went wrong to cause...?" At that point she would mention symptoms, lab reports, x-rays, etc. Then finally: "How do you fix it?" And thus it went with every case we discussed - very basic but a marvelous teaching method.

Often, Jane assigned me a case to work up and present back to her. This involved some study, which during an otherwise lackadaisical summer, I would never have done. No mercy was shown if she thought I had done a poor job. The woman was brilliant and for me to be ashamed of her company was beyond hypocrisy.

So the summer passed and with it a great experience. A farewell bash was attended by all the medical personnel at the Infirmary. Arthur Reynolds planned on staying at the Infirmary to complete his internship. The Irish contingent exchanged addresses; plans were made to get together during the course of the school year. My nurse friend and I shared a tearful farewell. Back to Dublin I went, considerably more knowledgeable, with an enhanced appreciation of Britain and its people.

(The sorrow my nurse-friend expressed at my departure had a short half-life. Sources reported that within the fortnight she had taken up with Dr. Reynolds. She always said that she would love a ride in his Alpha Romeo.)

The following year I heard Jane was back in Dublin for a visit. In an attempt to assuage my guilt and thank her, as I had just passed the Medicine exam, I made arrangements to meet her. We had dinner at Baileys, one of Dublin's finer restaurants; it was my first visit there.

During our conversation she mentioned that she had to return to China when she finished her contract at Wigan. Curious as to why, she explained that when she completed college in China she had taken a national exam, and as a result, was one of six in her province allowed to study abroad at government expense. There was a stipulation, however, that she return when studies had been completed. Her preference was to remain in the British Isles but if she did, the Chinese government would revoke her visa, notify the British authorities, and she would be extradited.

The evening finished with coffee and an after dinner drink during which we reminisced, and expressed our mutual fondness. A great meal was enjoyed as was the evening. My conscience was eased. After a hug and a kiss on the cheek, we said our good-byes. Although agreeing to stay in touch, we never did.

THE LOSS OF GOOD MEN

Shortly after returning, I was invited to a party by Doreen, the young lady from Earlsfort Terrace. Pat O'Brien came along and that evening met Frances, a friend of Doreen's, from Castletownbere in County Cork. She worked at the General Post Office in Dublin. Either entwined in dance or immersed in Guiness-fueled conversation, Pat, in a sweat-soaked white shirt, monopolized the young lady's attention for the remainder of the evening. At daybreak, a few of us found Mass at a church along the Liffey quays. Subsequent to the party, and to the consternation of many, Pat became irrationally smitten with this attractive female and under her influence acquired a heretofore unknown respectability and restraint. As a result, he withdrew from the pub scene, once his domain. Apparently he had found something more exciting than skittles.

Tom Lomas, after our apartment misadventure, had moved to the North side of Dublin and was also "doing a line" with a young lady. He, too, was conspicuously missing in action. Two stalwart chaps with great oat-sowing potential, fallen prey - and willingly, the story went - to the sway of the fairer sex. Many a pint was raised in commiseration for the loss of two good men.

My personal take on their co-option by the young ladies was mixed. It was comfortable to be assured of a little loving on a regular basis and abjure the rejections and dashed hopes that were the usual lot for the rest of us. But having suffered through all that and then one night to strike pay dirt, made the victory so much sweeter and less routine. I felt one's early twenties was not the time to be tethered to the same saddle, no matter how pleasant the ride. That and the fact that none of the women I knew ever indicated a desire to become more closely involved made my decision to remain with the boyos an easy one...

(After graduation Pat and Francis married, and in what certainly is a tribute to her patience, have remained so to this day. That chance meeting began a journey, which by my calculation, is approaching fifty years.)

The Final Push

The triumvirate of exams in OB/GYN, Medicine, and Surgery, were the major hurdles in the final clinical year. Also, when to sit the deferred Public Health exam, without jeopardizing chances of success in these major subjects, was my predicament.

Having finished obstetric rounds at Hollis Street one morning, I walked back to Surgeons with classmate, Neil O'Brien. Discussing my exam situation I mentioned that I had decided to focus on OB and let the Public Health slide until another time in the year. The major factor in the decision, I added, was that both exams were scheduled during the same week. Neil had a different take. The odds of failing both, he felt, was unlikely; even if one were failed, the situation wouldn't be much different than what it was presently. "Besides," he added, "you might get lucky and pass both."

Neil's advice was taken. The obstetrics paper wasn't bad: the orals were at the Coomb Hospital with Mr. DeValera. The take home feeling was it went well. Two days later I sat the Public Health exam. The paper was suspect but I fared better in the oral portion. Within a few days I learned both exams had been passed; finally I had caught up with the rest of the class.

I was, and am, amazed by the role chance plays in the path we eventually take in life. If I had not walked with Neil O'Brien that day I almost certainly would not have attempted the two exams. The result may have eventually been the same but who knows? If my Aunt Bertha hadn't gone to Europe that summer of 1955 and hadn't met someone in Scotland with a relative who attended the College of Surgeons, I never would have applied there. If the secretary in the Registrar's office hadn't been rude, I wouldn't have returned to find a more accommodating person. Chance encounters that impact generations.

Christmas day (I hoped my last in Dublin), was shared with Frank Swift and his family, who had invited me for dinner in their place over the pub. I felt privileged to have been asked to join in their celebration. Even at that time, 1960, Frank was looking forward to selling the business and enjoying retirement.

Although the economy was poor, pubs still brought a decent price; but nothing compared to their value a few years later when the Celtic Tiger found its voice. Hopefully he did well. (When I went back to Dublin some years later, the Toby Jug was gone, as were most of the adjoining buildings, replaced by a parking garage complex.)

With the Medicine exam scheduled for March, the new year, of necessity, demanded an increased emphasis on preparation. Hopefully my on-going investment since last year as a "disciple" of T.J. Ryan, a medical consultant I'd met at Jervis Street, would pay off. He was an excellent clinician, popular among students because of his exceptional teaching skills. T.J. often met after his private practice for the day, a consideration beyond what was expected of a consultant in a teaching hospital. As an adjunct to whatever topic he chose for discussion - e.g. diabetes, neurological disease - he had arranged, whenever possible, to have an in-patient with that condition available for discussion and examination. The allegiance was cemented by his guarantee that if we stuck with him and did the complementary studying, we would not only pass the medicine final but do so on our first attempt.

In this regard, the National Library on Kildare Street offered surroundings most conducive to study. An impressive portico fronted a wide atrium, from which a curved marble staircase ascended to the Reading Room. There, a vaulted ceiling enclosed a dimly lit, book-lined space, centered with rows of wooden desks symmetrically arranged, each with a green-shaded banker's light. Seldom crowded, a funeral-like silence, enforced by a formidable lady at the front desk, prevailed. Consistent in attendance were gray-haired gentlemen engrossed in their newspapers and scattered about, presumably involved in research, harried looking individuals surrounded by columns of ponderous appearing volumes. An afternoon of study was interrupted for a cigarette break on the portico or a cup of tea in the basement cafe across the street, managed by two elderly sisters.

By the time of the exam, with T.J.'s ramped up tutelage and that of Jane in Wigan, I felt well prepared for a change. The effort was rewarded as I passed quite handily, as did all of T.J.'s "boys." In appreciation of his expert coaching, we chipped in for a gift - a bottle of Jameson whiskey.

During this time, more by coincidence than design, a relationship developed with Bernie Lavelle, a student nurse I had met during my clerkship at Jervis Street. Initial impressions were formed in the break room above the operating rooms: a brunette of medium height, nice smile, and mischievous eyes; her OR garb prevented further observations. Additional conversations in morning medical clinics revealed a sharp sense of humor laced with sarcasm and a hint of interest. Needing an escort, Bernie invited me to a hospital-sponsored formal dance at the Gresham Hotel, which went well. Beyond that, a few movies and the occasional dance were the extent of our dating. Friendly enough, I guess, because an invitation was extended to visit, for a weekend, her and her family at their home on Achill Island in County Mayo. My acceptance was prompt.

The Lavelles, I learned, were quite prominent in the area, involved in various enterprises, including a pub which remains to this day. I met various members of the family, whose company I thoroughly enjoyed.

Saturday night we attended a local dance. Diminished by a large stage, a four-piece ensemble provided the music. The men, all spiffed up in white shirts and jackets, lined one wall; the women, cloistered in conversation, the opposite. Bernie knew many of them, mainly sons and daughters of local farmers. The music was mostly British and American pop tunes: the Beatles and the Rolling Stones not yet on the scene. Lonnie Donegan's skiffle tunes, Frank Sinatra and Pat Boone's ballads, and a little rock and roll were the musical mainstays of the evening. Our bodies fit nicely when we danced, tentatively touching, her cheek against mine. Alcohol wasn't served but it became apparent, as the night progressed, that an alternate source had been found.

I found out later that Bernie, being with a "Yank," became

fodder for local gossip, some of which wasn't complementary. Americans, it was assumed by many, were wealthy, with a singular intent regarding the fairer sex: any woman who consorted with one must be "putting out." Scarcely beyond the hand-holding stage, neither criterion applied at that time in our relationship. Comfortable with each other, there was a niggling suspicion, that if the liaison were to continue, it might develop into something more.

After Mass the following morning, Bernie packed lunches and we explored the island in the family's second car. Clumps of white cloud scudded across a blue sky as we made our way out of town. Bernie pointed out, on a distant hill, the former residence of Captain Boycott, an English landlord so despised by his tenants that they refused to work for him; the townspeople denied him services. Their actions introduced the verb "boycott" into the vernacular. We also passed by the cottage where the author Graham Greene lived for a period of time with his Irish mistress, and when not otherwise engaged, worked on his novel, *The Heart of the Matter*.

Soon the few villages were left behind and we found ourselves in a beautiful but barren landscape, its scant vegetation blown brown by the salt of Atlantic winds. Traveling the Atlantic Drive we followed the jagged coastline, tracking in-land on occasion through rock-strewn tracts of land and low-lying mountains, soon hooking back to the coast and the vast shimmering sea. Sheep were noted on the foothills but not on the higher elevations. "It's the wind," Bernie explained. "They'd be blown away, and the good grass is gone, so they wouldn't survive."

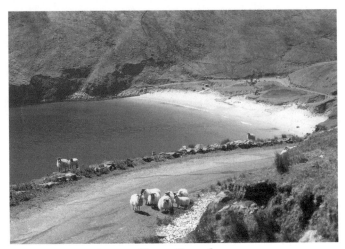

Keem Strand

Further west, we walked Keem Strand, a horse-shoe shaped beach at the head of a wide bay, enclosed on either side by imposing cliffs. Two young boys, pant legs rolled up, were wading in the water. We found the perfect place for lunch. At the far end of the beach stood a derelict rescue station, walls smashed through, large portions of roof missing, but with a solid seawall to lean against.

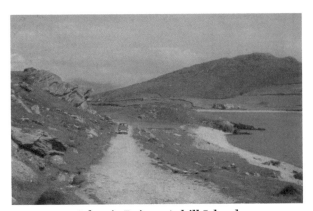

Atlantic Drive - Achill Island

Calm waters soundlessly lapped the shore, while in the distance, beyond the bay's entrance, the wave-ridden Atlantic churned. Our conversation was lazy: small talk about Jervis St., the dance the previous night, local history, her family. We held hands. In the sun her hair had gained an auburn burnish.

"Could you ever imagine living in Ireland?" she asked.

I shrugged my shoulders. "I think, Bernie, if I didn't have a family expecting me home, I'd stay."

"And will you not be coming back?" She turned to me. "Ah do, Gene, before it's all forgotten, before you're all caught up in America."

"There's no doubt I'll be coming back; it's when, I don't know." I smiled and shook my head. "But I'm getting ahead of myself, Bernie, I've still got an exam to get through."

"Oh, you'll do fine."

"What makes you so sure?"

"I've appealed to a higher power." She laughed, then added, "And I've never been denied."

Bernie started to put the lunch leftovers in the basket. I added the drink bottles to the collection on the dirt floor of the building.

Walking back to the car, she stopped and turned to me. Her face, caught between shadow and sun, was beautiful. "Wasn't going to tell you," she began, "but about three weeks ago I made a weekend retreat. You know, you can dedicate a retreat for certain intentions, don't you?"

"No, I didn't know."

"Well, you can. So at the start of the weekend I made three petitions. First, that you pass your exams." She smiled. "That's the easy one. Second, that you'll be happy in your life as a doctor." She started to walk away.

"And the third?" I asked.

"Oh, that one I'll keep to myself, if you don't mind."

In the current lexicon I was totally "blown away" by what I thought was an extraordinarily generous thing to do, for someone she hardly knew. I thanked her - and have continued to thank her at every Mass I've attended since.

From Keem Strand we continued to Achill Head which was, Bernie insisted, the closest point in Ireland to America. A moss-covered promontory fell away to sheer cliff, at the bottom of which angry Atlantic rollers roiled against the first obstruction encountered in their journey. Birds darted in and out of crevices on the rock face. The winds had swept clean all vegetation except some low-lying bushes, their branches speckled white. As far as one could see along the jagged coastline, not another person or evidence of habitation could be seen.

"Spectacular!" I shouted to Bernie over the wind. She smiled and nodded.

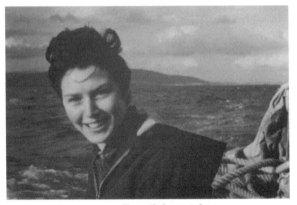

Bernie Lavelle off the Irish Coast

As we turned to leave, I brought her to me and parting hair blown across her face, kissed her. Tentative to start, her lips were soon soft, full, and lingering. Walking back to the car, I turned for a last look.

"Bernie," I said, "we must come back to this very spot one day." She said nothing but took my hand. (And one day, we did.)

Mrs. Lavelle made up a lunch for my return to Dublin. Sincere thanks were extended to the family for their hospitality; Bernie drove me to the train station in Westport. Our goodbyes were casual. "Let's keep in touch," I offered. She agreed that we should. In my compartment, I pulled down the window and waved back to her on the platform. A white handkerchief fluttered as she raised her hand in response.

(It would be another three years before our paths would cross again, and the story would not have a fairy-tale ending.)

W ith the end in sight and not wanting to spend another five months in Dublin, preparation for the Surgery exam assumed an added urgency. During this same period, I took the ECFMG exam, with about a dozen others, in a room at the American Embassy. It was a requirement for all foreign medical graduates who wished to practice in the United States.

Surgery as a specialty generated little interest for me, partially because of the mechanical skills required. Manual dexterity was not, and is not, my strong suit. I had great respect and not a little jealousy, for those who possessed those skills. Also, I didn't think our Professor of Surgery, Mr. J. Seton Pringle, was a particularly inspiring teacher.

The exam consisted of a written portion, an oral (conducted before two or three surgeons), and an in-hospital clinical evaluation. In this section, students would obtain a history, complete a physical examination, review lab and x-ray reports, and then present findings, diagnosis, and a treatment plan for their assigned patient.

The day of reckoning arrived. The ten to twelve questions on the written portion I felt I handled well. The oral was scheduled for the following morning at 9:00 a.m. After an interminable wait outside the oral exam room, the door finally opened. As the student leaving passed, she whispered "diverticulitis."

A bank of x-ray-viewing boxes were lined up behind three examiners seated at a broad, brown table stacked with folders. Taking turns, they asked a series of questions, a large number of which concerned the x-rays. Based on the occasional nod, I felt I was doing well. Finally, one asked, "And what do you think we have for a diagnosis here."

The moment of truth. Although not my first inclination, I

hesitantly answered, "Diverticulitis."

An "oh, really?" expression came on their collective faces, and as if in unison, they shifted in their seats and leaned forward on the table. "Tell me about diverticulitis," one prompted. And another said, "Show me where you see that on the x-ray." The questions continued as to how I arrived at this increasingly apparent, wrong diagnosis. My shirt was sticking to me. Then they paused.

Glances were exchanged between them. "Anyone have anything else?" asked the surgeon seated at the center. No response was forthcoming. "Then," he added, "just one more from me: What else do you think it could be?" The options I offered were met with blank stares. Finally, mercifully, the same surgeon announced: "You're dismissed."

Any hope I had of passing, I realized, had vanished. My clinical exam was scheduled for that afternoon at the Richmond Hospital. *Why waste my time and theirs?* I thought. Chalk it up to a bad day; repeat the exam in the fall.

Leaving the college I headed toward Grafton Street. As I was about to turn onto King Street and the Toby, I stopped to light a cigarette. In the distance, I heard my name being called. There, on the opposite corner, was Neil O'Brien heading to his oral. Joining me he asked how I had done. I related my experience - so horrendous, I added, that I had decided not to do the clinical portion that afternoon. Neil thought this was foolish; he felt I should give it a go.

"What'n the hell have you got to lose?" was his parting shot.

He was right before, maybe... Back at the digs, I read through some notes, then headed to Saint Kevins, the Catholic church across the street. The place was empty. Kneeling at the altar rail, I prayed for help. If I passed, I promised to do a retreat at Loch Derg, considered the toughest retreat house in Ireland. With that bargain established, I took a bus into Dublin and another to the Richmond Hospital.

The case assigned was pretty straight-forward: an osteomy-elitis of the leg in an elderly man. Dr. Leonard Abrahamson was the examiner. A medical attending, he was probably involved because surgery had been completed, the remaining treatment primarily medical. Dr. Abrahamson enjoyed a reputation for being a tough examiner who delighted in intimidation. After presenting my history and physical exam, he questioned me re-garding the pathology, the reasons for surgery, the surgery in-volved, and the medical treatment. No comments were made during the course of my responses, which I didn't consider a good sign.

Eventually, he did string a few sentences together, mainly to inform me that my presentation was not only inadequate but dangerous to the patient.

Specifically, he noted that the dosage of the antibiotic (Pen-icillin) I had suggested was "too large with an elderly patient like this; it could kill him." The doctor appeared impatient and anxious to leave.

I figured I had one last shot. "Sir," I responded, "I read re-cently in a medical journal that larger doses of antibiotics were becoming necessary in osteomyelitis."

"Really?" said Dr. Abrahamson. "And why is that?" His tone was patronizing.

"Bacterial resistance, the article said. The bacteria have found ways to block the antibiotic from working."

"And I suppose the dose you suggested is what's recom-mended?" he said, eyeing me closely.

"As far as I remember, Sir."

For a few seconds he looked at me. "What's the name of the journal?"

I told him I had forgotten.

"But you are certain you read it?" he asked. He must have known as well as I that it was pure fiction - but then again, may-be he wasn't sure.

"Yes, Sir," I answered firmly. The doctor seemed about to make another comment but turned and walked away.

Later that day, a fellow student, Sean Hannigan, somehow obtained the list of those who had failed the clinical portion that day. My name wasn't on it. Two days later I officially learned I had passed Surgery. The telegram I sent to my father was signed, "Doc."

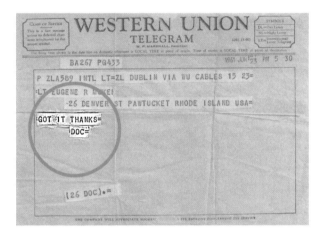

DEBT PAID

I made plans to get home. One problem, still unresolved, was my debt to Joe McGrath. One hundred and fifty Irish pounds were owed, about $450.00 - an unheard of sum for a student to owe a pub. Joe never threatened to cut me off, but he did remind me, now and then, that it was getting a little heavy.

Ben Healy, an American doing medicine at the University of Cork, paid me a visit around that time. Through high school we had lived on the same street in Pawtucket, R.I. In conversation, I mentioned my indebtedness. Ben suggested that I contact Memorial Hospital in Pawtucket. They were looking for interns, and he felt certain they would lend me the money, if I indicated my intent to work there. I promptly wrote a letter and in a matter of days, received an acceptance into their intern program and a check for $500.00. The dollars were promptly changed to pounds, and probably to the amazement of Joe McGrath, I paid my bill in full.

(However, two other debts remain to this day, and in a nod to honesty, are herewith noted: the $500.00 loan from Memorial Hospital has not been paid, and the promise made to the baby Jesus at the altar rail of St. Kevin's - to make a retreat at Loch Derg- has not been honored. In the former instance, I could rationalize that they got their money's worth and then some, but that's beside the point. In the latter instance, hopefully the guilt I've carried around these years, has been duly noted by whomever keeps score in these matters; and of course, there's still time to make things right!)

While in the confessional mode, another matter requires revision: the victory in ping-pong previously described. In truth, the red-headed twelve-year-old, cast and all, whipped my butt good

– real good. His total domination was almost as embarrassing as his offer of lessons. Adding a bogus triumph to an already suspect athletic resume seems unbecoming in an otherwise reasonably credible memoir. So, after consideration, I've withdrawn my claim to the table tennis championship; my conscience now clear.

T he graduation was a splendid affair. Matt O'Connor, our pathology professor, was to present the diplomas. Formally attired in our graduation gowns, we sat in the main hall of the College. All in great form, we waited for the proceedings to begin.

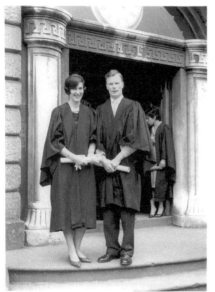 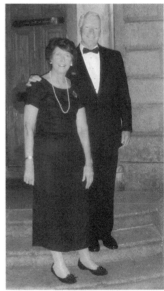

Graduation Day with Classmate
Colette Pegum and Fifty Years Later

The College porter, Maxwell, attired like a Sergeant-at-Arms, appeared and passed a note to me. It indicated that I hadn't paid the Conferring fee. Without payment, he indicated, I would not receive a diploma. Although a relatively small amount, five pounds as I recollect, I didn't have it with me. In what seems to be a metaphor for my college experience, a collection was taken up, the required sum accumulated, and brought to Maxwell. Des McManus, sitting beside me, was the major contributor with a pound note. With the final toll paid and the hearty handshake of Matt O'Connor, I became the first graduate of the Royal College of Surgeons from the United States. And lest we forget, made possible by a pack of Lucky Strike cigarettes and a young lady willing to bend the rules.

My farewell tour would not have been complete without hooking up with Dan Savage one last time. Since leaving the digs I hadn't seen him. Miss Halligan mentioned that he had stopped by a couple times. On one visit she learned that his wife, Anne, had lost a baby. They both were very distraught for an extended period. But as of his last visit, Miss Halligan felt they had come to terms with the loss: Anne had returned to her job at Cleary's; Dan seemed like his old self. I called Dan and we arranged to meet.

Their flat, located in the Templeogue area of Dublin, was in a former factory that had been refurbished and converted to apartments. Their place, on the third level, was at the end of a long corridor, redolent of a variety of cooking smells, and lit with a series of harsh fluorescent lights. Dan, thinner than I remembered, welcomed me with a handshake, his wife, on the phone, with a nod. The flat, although small, "suited them just fine," Dan said. With a wave he indicated the location of the bedroom, bathroom, and kitchenette. The larger room, centered by a wooden table, served as both the living room and dining area; light was provided by a single unshaded bulb at the end of a cord dangling from the ceiling.

I had brought a few bottles of stout. As we sipped, reminiscences flowed: the days in the digs, the characters who passed through and the "gas" times that were had.

"One more time, Dan. Do the Four Farrellys," I requested.

He began, but quite abruptly, stopped half-way through. "Not the same, not the right setting," he said. And it was true. The room, bare except for the table and chairs, its unadorned walls cast in shadows, was indeed dismal.

Rather awkwardly, we said our good-byes. His wife gave me a kiss on the cheek and asked me to stay in touch. Dan shook my hand. "Don't forget old Ireland." He turned away. "For, Ireland," his voice seemed to break a bit, "won't be forgetting you."

Miss Halligan was happy for my success. Except for some short absences, my entire time in Dublin was with her. Through the good and bad times, hangovers, exams failed and passed, and the occasional illness, she was there. Many were the Saturday nights, having stumbled up the stairs heading to bed, when her voice beckoned from the kitchen, "Like a bite to eat, Mr. McKee?" Miss Halligan always left a meal for Joe, for his return from second shift at the newspaper. From whatever had been prepared - tripe with a cream sauce and boiled potatoes come to mind - she made up a plate for me. She lent me money and toward the end of my stay did my laundry.

As far as I was able to determine, aside from the week at Christmas, she never took vacations. Not married, there was no evidence of a male interest. I only saw her dressed up on one occasion - to attend a funeral. Mass was seldom missed, the first offered each Sunday. Aside from the occasional party in the kitchen with the house "regulars," she had no social life. Her day began around 5:00 a.m. and no matter what time I came in at night, the light was always on.

We said our goodbyes in the kitchen.

"You've been a wonderful tenant, Mr. McKee. I hope everything goes well back in the States," she said.

"You've brought me luck, Miss Halligan. That's the reason I stayed all these years," I said, then added, "It certainly wasn't the food," which got a laugh from her. I gave her a hug. "Thanks for everything you've done."

"I'll miss you, Mr. McKee. God Bless."

(In the spring of 1982, I visited Ireland with my family whom she was delighted to meet. She told them something of the old days at Hyde House, how the clientele had changed. "Don't get them like your father, Mr. O'Brien, and Mr. McLaughlin anymore," she told the kids, "real gentlemen they were." Miss Halligan also mentioned that Dan and his wife had returned to Galway and that Frank Gillan had died some years earlier from a cancer of the throat. She appeared even smaller than I remembered. Crippled with arthritis, she was failing. Two years later she died. A wonderful lady - remembered fondly.)

THE LAST TOAST

My last hours in Dublin were spent at the Toby Jug with Tom Lomas and Frank Swift. While Tom and I reminisced about the great years we'd had, Frank recollected the "gas" nights in the Toby. Totally bereft of decent clothes for my return, Pat O'Brien had given me a jacket, a shirt and a pair of shoes for the trip, a veneer of respectability in keeping with my newly acquired professional status. The only problem: Pat reached 6' 4 with a decent frame, while I was 6'1 and skinny. (Some days later, arriving at Union Station in Providence, Bertha on seeing me, erupted in gales of laughter. Between gusts she managed, "You look...just like... Charlie Chaplin...")

Then the time came to catch the 2:00 p.m. train from Kingsbridge to Cork. Frank called a cab, closed the pub, and we headed off. As we threaded our way down Grafton Street, past Trinity College, over the O'Connell Bridge and the Liffey River, past Jervis Street and the Rotunda Hospital, I tried to fix the image of each in my mind.

Goodbyes were made on the platform. Frank's handshake included a couple of baby Power whiskeys slipped into my jacket. My last image of Dublin: waving back to Frank, still in his bar apron, and Tom.

Off to Cobh, having finished a journey that began in 1955. My Aunt Bertha's "project" that had offered scant hope of success, ended with a piece of paper that opened the door to another adventure - a medical career in the United States.

Five years hadn't changed the Dublin of my recollection, the old haunts: Roberts Cafe, Bewleys, Davy Byrnes were all intact. Joe Dwyer had sold his place on Leeson Street; the Toby Jug remained but Frank Swift, I was told, was ailing.

Walking down Harcourt Street, toward Stephens Green, I saw a woman coming toward me, pushing a pram, a small child trailing behind. Her long skirt brushed the pavement and a shawl, draped over her shoulder, partially obscured her face. As I passed, she called to the child who lagged behind. The profile seemed familiar.

"Nora."

The woman looked up, shielding her eyes from the sun.

"Good God, if it ain't the Yank."

"And I almost passed you by."

"Well I ain't the young thing you knew back in Jervo, you know."

Her face was weathered and more tan than I remembered but the fine features remained. She stayed stooped, bent over the handle of the pram.

"I've often wondered about you, Nora. So how've you been?"

"Well, I ain't in the headlines, Yank, but I married a boyo from Jacobs and got me two kids. We're getting along. And ya-self?"

"Working in a military hospital. Will be out in about a year and then we'll see what happens."

Nora seemed uncomfortable, rolling the pram back and forth with scarcely a look toward me. Awkwardly we chatted, pauses rescued by small talk of her children and family. "Yeh, Ma still has the cart on Camden Street." When I inquired after her father she merely shrugged her shoulders.

Nora leaned toward the pram. "I have to go. The baby..."

"Nora," I interrupted, "there's something that's bothered me all this time."

"What's that?"

"That Thanksgiving when you invited me, and I never turned up. I never explained..."

"Oh, that," she said. Moving to the side of the pram, she fussed with the baby, tucking in the blankets. "That's awhile back, Yank. I've almost forgotten. Surprised you remember." Her voice, raised against the noise of the traffic seemed raspy.

"I've felt badly, Nora; never thought I'd see you again...to apologize."

"Don't be sorry. I was a right ol' fool to expect you. When I told Ma ya'd promised, she just laughed. 'Too fancy for the likes of us,' she said."

"That's not true."

"As I remember," she went on, "ya didn't miss much. The feckin' bird wasn't cooked right and we all ended up in a pub getting shit faced. Even Pa, still in his shirt and tie, all dressed up for the big event." Nora shook her head. "The neighbors thought I made ya up in me head. A big joke it was."

"I'm sorry, Nora."

Nora turned, pulled the shawl back and looked at me, full in the face. "You hurt me terrible, Yank." She paused. "But no harm. Water under the bridge, as they say."

"Nora," I began. She shook her head. She didn't want to hear anymore.

The boy at her side tugged at her skirt. She nodded and told him they were leaving. About to push away, she hesitated. "By the way," she said, "D'ya remember the woman in the ward that night?"

"Of course."

"She passed away last week."

"How do you know?"

"After the hospital we stayed friends. Matter of fact, she was

Donal's godmother," she said, nodding toward the boy at her side. "She knew ya were with me that night. Never let on."

"I'll be damned."

"Anyway, she said if I ever saw ya to say thanks... so I am." She took the little boy's hand and turned toward me. "Bye, Yank. Take care of yaself."

"Nora, let me give you something...for the kids," I said, reaching for my wallet.

Her look was total disdain. "I don't take no feck'n charity."

I watched as she crossed the street and continued down the other side. At the corner, she stopped to light a cigarette. A bus passed; when I looked again, Nora was gone.

POSTSCRIPT

A s one in the fourth quarter of life's game, hoping for an overtime or two, a broad vista is available for review. The sweep of events is more easily cataloged into segments of relative importance - school, profession, marriage, military, children - the forest tangle now a neater grove of trees. With this narrowed prism, the highlight reel for my 20's would be, without question, my time abroad, and more specifically, Dublin and Surgeons. The experience, an abridged version of which is offered in this memoir, began as a lark, and other than brief periods of concentration, continued as a lark. Unshackled from the constraints and discipline of home and school, for the first time I was free to do what I liked with no one to answer to - a liberating experience. The splendid romp of student life, not weighted with significant concerns or responsibilities - aside from a few bumps, detours and wrong turns along the way - flowed unperturbed. Bolstered by youth, good health, and an ever-hovering guardian angel - whom I hope to thank one day - the story ended well.

And as much a part of my education in Dublin as Surgeons, were the years spent at Hyde House and on South Circular Road. The digs offered a unique vantage to meet, observe and converse with an endless stream of personalities. Briefly joined on their journey, they comprised an eclectic group: each with a story, baggage, and ambition. Diverse characters from different sections of the country all had something to offer, be it background, idiosyncrasies, intelligence, humor or just their take on life - a cultural montage of Ireland in the 50s and early 60s.

On occasion, I'm asked questions relative to my Gaelic experience: Did I have any regrets doing medicine in Ireland? If the same conditions prevailed would I do it again? Did I think the training was equivalent to that offered in the U.S.?

In response to the first queries, I have absolutely no regrets about doing my training in Ireland and in similar circumstances would do so again. The opportunity to live in another country, have a chance to absorb the culture, and appreciate the beauty of the environment and its people, was a unique experience. Other physicians I know who have trained overseas have voiced similar opinions.

The decision not to accept the slot offered at New York Medical College was based ostensibly on economics. And certainly that was the case - loans would have been needed. Years later I asked my Aunt Bertha what she was thinking when pushing me into medicine with no way to pay the freight. She casually answered, "I would have mortgaged the house."

My God, I thought, *how fortunate it never happened.* To be in that competitive environment - with a house ransomed so you could be there - would have created unimaginable pressure.

But also, I was happy where I was. Friends had been made and something about the Irish way, the relaxed attitude, suited me. If I had to do something in which I had little interest, at least I got to do it in a place I enjoyed.

Relative to the merits of the two educational systems, I have no firsthand knowledge of the American system. However, having worked with many American-trained physicians over the years, I've drawn conclusions. The medical schools in the U.S. were/are the best in the world, and no question: only the most qualified gain acceptance to them. Comparing our first year class to a similar one in the States, there was little doubt that the Americans were academically superior at that juncture. But I would maintain that as the curriculum continued, attrition took the toll of those not cutting it - the wheat from the chaff, if you will. In my class at Surgeons we lost approximately 40% of our medical group by the time of graduation. The U.S. schools' attrition rate was around 5%; admission standards being such that if you were smart enough to get in the place, you were smart enough to get out. The students who received their medical degrees from Surgeons in 1961, I submit, were as well prepared as their counterparts graduating in the States.

But something I can reasonably reference were their respective capabilities in the actual practice of medicine. Over the years, I've worked with and supervised many physicians in various settings - hospital, private practice, military, and industrial; some trained abroad, others in the U.S. A generalization (always a risky business): I contend that the Yanks prevailed in academics; the foreign-trained students had the edge on the clinical side...just my opinion.

In today's world, technology has significantly leveled the playing field. The major medical institutions world-wide are equivalent in the expertise brought to the patient. Detection of disease has become largely machine and lab driven; the day of the bed-side diagnosis - the laying on of hands – largely a ritual of another time. These observations are not offered as the rant of a wistful curmudgeon (who utilizes these marvelous modalities on a regular basis), but rather as a tip of the hat to those who accomplished so much with so little.

The running of the years enhances recollection: the grand times become grander, the bad days hardly remembered - a pot-holed piece of highway paved smooth. And so it is with me. Nothing remains but the best of memories. Along with Humphrey and Ingrid, who in *Casablanca* always had Paris, I will, God help me, always have Dublin.

Through the ensuing decades, questions tucked in dark recesses periodically surfaced. What if I had been allowed my own academic choices back in the Holy Cross days? Where would that road have led? Would I have discovered a passion or merely a different job that would also have provided a comfortable living? These queries do not imply regret, but rather speculation as to what might have been found along the path not taken. So a curiosity remains: of a song never sung, of a race never run.

And here I sit, fifty years later, typing this recollection - still practicing medicine...who knew!!!

E.B. McKee, MD
May 2013

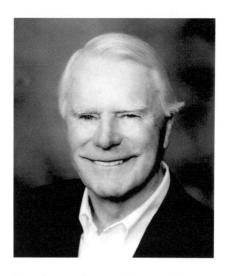

After graduation from the College of Surgeons in 1961, Dr. McKee completed an internship and residency in Family Medicine at Memorial Hospital in Pawtucket R.I. Then, fulfilling an ROTC commitment, he entered the US Air Force, and was assigned to the 551st USAF Hospital at Otis AFB on Cape Cod, Mass., as a General Medical Officer. Subsequently he was chosen to attend the School of Aerospace Medicine in San Antonio, Texas. Upon completion of that program he returned to Otis AFB where he headed the Flight Surgeons office. Discharged from active military duty in 1966, he joined the medical staff of United Airlines working in Denver; Washington, D.C; and New York. (Dr. McKee maintained a military affiliation and retired, after twenty years of service, as Hospital Commander of the 143rd Airlift Wing, R. I. Air National Guard.)

Dr. McKee returned to R.I. in 1970 and established a family practice, became board certified, and maintained the practice until 2000. During this time-span he also directed the occupational health program at the Electric Boat Division of General Dynamics in R.I.

Upon retirement from private practice, Dr. McKee was ap-

pointed Medical Director of an urgent care facility, a position maintained until 2010. He continues to provide services at the facility, albeit with a modified schedule.

Dr. McKee has occupied various executive and clinical leadership positions at South County Hospital in Wakefield, R.I., and he has enjoyed associations with various medical and civic organizations over the years. He is a member of the R.I. Air National Guard Society, Mensa, and the R.I. Historical Society. Married and the father of five, Dr. McKee presently resides in Narragansett, R.I. Author contact: genem1@cox.net